ADOLESCENCE

GENERAL EDITORS

Dale C. Garell, M.D.
Medical Director, California Children Services, Department of Health
  Services, County of Los Angeles
Associate Dean for Curriculum
Clinical Professor, Department of Pediatrics & Family Medicine,
  University of Southern California School of Medicine
Former President, Society for Adolescent Medicine

Solomon H. Snyder, M.D.
Distinguished Service Professor of Neuroscience, Pharmacology, and
  Psychiatry, Johns Hopkins University School of Medicine
Former president, Society of Neuroscience
Albert Lasker Award in Medical Research, 1978

CONSULTING EDITORS

Robert W. Blum, M.D., Ph.D.
Associate Professor, School of Public Health and Department of
  Pediatrics
Director, Adolescent Health Program, University of Minnesota
Consultant, World Health Organization

Charles E. Irwin, Jr., M.D.
Associate Professor of Pediatrics; Director, Division of Adolescent
  Medicine, University of California, San Francisco

Lloyd J. Kolbe, Ph.D.
Chief, Office of School Health & Special Projects, Center for Health
  Promotion & Education, Centers for Disease Control
President, American School Health Association

Jordan J. Popkin
Director, Division of Federal Employee Occupational Health, U.S. Public
  Health Service Region I

Joseph L. Rauh, M.D.
Professor of Pediatrics and Medicine, Adolescent Medicine, Children's
  Hospital Medical Center, Cincinnati
Former president, Society for Adolescent Medicine

THE ENCYCLOPEDIA OF

H E A L T H

THE LIFE CYCLE

Dale C. Garell, M.D. · General Editor

ADOLESCENCE

Rebecca Stefoff

Introduction by C. Everett Koop, M.D., Sc.D.
former Surgeon General, U.S. Public Health Service

CHELSEA HOUSE PUBLISHERS
New York · Philadelphia

The goal of the ENCYCLOPEDIA OF HEALTH *is to provide general information in the ever-changing areas of physiology, psychology, and related medical issues. The titles in this series are not intended to take the place of the professional advice of a physician or other health care professional.*

Chelsea House Publishers
EDITOR-IN-CHIEF Remmel Nunn
MANAGING EDITOR Karyn Gullen Browne
COPY CHIEF Juliann Barbato
PICTURE EDITOR Adrian G. Allen
ART DIRECTOR Maria Epes
DEPUTY COPY CHIEF Mark Rifkin
ASSISTANT ART DIRECTOR Loraine Machlin
MANUFACTURING MANAGER Gerald Levine
SYSTEMS MANAGER Rachel Vigier
PRODUCTION MANAGER Joseph Romano
PRODUCTION COORDINATOR Marie Claire Cebrián

The Encyclopedia of Health
SENIOR EDITOR Paula Edelson

Staff for ADOLESCENCE
ASSISTANT EDITOR Jennifer Fleissner
EDITORIAL ASSISTANT Leigh Hope Wood
PICTURE RESEARCHER Villette Harris
SENIOR DESIGNER Marjorie Zaum
DESIGN ASSISTANT Debora Smith

3 5 7 9 8 6 4 2

Library of Congress Cataloging-in-Publication Data

Stefoff, Rebecca
  Adolescence/Rebecca Stefoff.
    p. cm.—(The Encyclopedia of health)
  Includes bibliographical references.
  Summary: Describes the biological and psychological changes that
occur during adolescence and examines social problems, questions,
and adjustments that are part of the transition from childhood to
adulthood.
  ISBN 0-7910-0033-8
       0-7910-0473-2 (pbk.)
  1. Adolescence—Juvenile literature. [1. Adolescence.]
I. Title. II. Series.   89-48522
HQ796.S8245 1990   CIP
305.2'35—dc20   AC

CONTENTS

PREVENTION AND EDUCATION: THE KEYS TO GOOD HEALTH

C. Everett Koop, M.D., Sc.D.
former Surgeon General,
U.S. Public Health Service

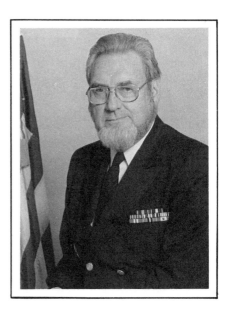

The issue of health education has received particular attention in recent years because of the presence of AIDS in the news. But our response to this particular tragedy points up a number of broader issues that doctors, public health officials, educators, and the public face. In particular, it points up the necessity for sound health education for citizens of all ages.

Over the past 25 years this country has been able to bring about dramatic declines in the death rates for heart disease, stroke, accidents, and, for people under the age of 45, cancer. Today, Americans generally eat better and take better care of themselves than ever before. Thus, with the help of modern science and technology, they have a better chance of surviving serious—even catastrophic—illnesses. That's the good news.

But, like every phonograph record, there's a flip side, and one with special significance for young adults. According to a report issued in 1979 by Dr. Julius Richmond, my predecessor as Surgeon General, Americans aged 15 to 24 had a higher death rate in 1979 than they did 20 years earlier. The causes: violent death and injury, alcohol and drug abuse, unwanted pregnancies, and sexually transmitted diseases. Adolescents are particularly vulnerable because they are beginning to explore their own sexuality and perhaps to experiment with drugs. The need for educating young people is critical, and the price of neglect is high.

Yet even for the population as a whole, our health is still far from what it could be. Why? A 1974 Canadian government report attributed all death and disease to four broad elements: inadequacies in

7

the health care system, behavioral factors or unhealthy life-styles, environmental hazards, and human biological factors.

To be sure, there are diseases that are still beyond the control of even our advanced medical knowledge and techniques. And despite yearnings that are as old as the human race itself, there is no "fountain of youth" to ward off aging and death. Still, there is a solution to many of the problems that undermine sound health. In a word, that solution is prevention. Prevention, which includes health promotion and education, saves lives, improves the quality of life, and, in the long run, saves money.

In the United States, organized public health activities and preventive medicine have a long history. Important milestones include the improvement of sanitary procedures and the development of pasteurized milk in the late 19th century, and the introduction in the mid-20th century of effective vaccines against polio, measles, German measles, mumps, and other once-rampant diseases. Internationally, organized public health efforts began on a wide-scale basis with the International Sanitary Conference of 1851, to which 12 nations sent representatives. The World Health Organization, founded in 1948, continues these efforts under the aegis of the United Nations, with particular emphasis on combatting communicable diseases and the training of health care workers.

Despite these accomplishments, much remains to be done in the field of prevention. For too long, we have had a medical care system that is science- and technology-based, focused, essentially, on illness and mortality. It is now patently obvious that both the social and the economic costs of such a system are becoming insupportable.

Implementing prevention—and its corollaries, health education and promotion—is the job of several groups of people.

First, the medical and scientific professions need to continue basic scientific research, and here we are making considerable progress. But increased concern with prevention will also have a decided impact on how primary care doctors practice medicine. With a shift to health-based rather than morbidity-based medicine, the role of the "new physician" will include a healthy dose of patient education.

Second, practitioners of the social and behavioral sciences—psychologists, economists, city planners—along with lawyers, business leaders, and government officials—must solve the practical and ethical dilemmas confronting us: poverty, crime, civil rights, literacy, education, employment, housing, sanitation, environmental protection, health care delivery systems, and so forth. All of these issues affect public health.

Third is the public at large. We'll consider that very important group in a moment.

Fourth, and the linchpin in this effort, is the public health profession—doctors, epidemiologists, teachers—who must harness the professional expertise of the first two groups and the common sense and cooperation of the third, the public. They must define the problems statistically and qualitatively and then help us set priorities for finding the solutions.

To a very large extent, improving those statistics is the responsibility of every individual. So let's consider more specifically what the role of the individual should be and why health education is so important to that role. First, and most obviously, individuals can protect themselves from illness and injury and thus minimize their need for professional medical care. They can eat nutritious food, get adequate exercise, avoid tobacco, alcohol, and drugs, and take prudent steps to avoid accidents. The proverbial "apple a day keeps the doctor away" is not so far from the truth, after all.

Second, individuals should actively participate in their own medical care. They should schedule regular medical and dental checkups. Should they develop an illness or injury, they should know when to treat themselves and when to seek professional help. To gain the maximum benefit from any medical treatment that they do require, individuals must become partners in that treatment. For instance, they should understand the effects and side effects of medications. I counsel young physicians that there is no such thing as too much information when talking with patients. But the corollary is the patient must know enough about the nuts and bolts of the healing process to understand what the doctor is telling him. That is at least partially the patient's responsibility.

Education is equally necessary for us to understand the ethical and public policy issues in health care today. Sometimes individuals will encounter these issues in making decisions about their own treatment or that of family members. Other citizens may encounter them as jurors in medical malpractice cases. But we all become involved, indirectly, when we elect our public officials, from school board members to the president. Should surrogate parenting be legal? To what extent is drug testing desirable, legal, or necessary? Should there be public funding for family planning, hospitals, various types of medical research, and medical care for the indigent? How should we allocate scant technological resources, such as kidney dialysis and organ transplants? What is the proper role of government in protecting the rights of patients?

What are the broad goals of public health in the United States today? In 1980, the Public Health Service issued a report aptly entitled *Promoting Health—Preventing Disease: Objectives for the Nation.* This report expressed its goals in terms of mortality and in terms of intermediate goals in education and health improvement. It identified 15 major concerns: controlling high blood pressure; improving family planning; improving pregnancy care and infant health; increasing the rate of immunization; controlling sexually transmitted diseases; controlling the presence of toxic agents and radiation in the environment; improving occupational safety and health; preventing accidents; promoting water fluoridation and dental health; controlling infectious diseases; decreasing smoking; decreasing alcohol and drug abuse; improving nutrition; promoting physical fitness and exercise; and controlling stress and violent behavior.

For healthy adolescents and young adults (ages 15 to 24), the specific goal was a 20% reduction in deaths, with a special focus on motor vehicle injuries and alcohol and drug abuse. For adults (ages 25 to 64), the aim was 25% fewer deaths, with a concentration on heart attacks, strokes, and cancers.

Smoking is perhaps the best example of how individual behavior can have a direct impact on health. Today cigarette smoking is recognized as the most important single preventable cause of death in our society. It is responsible for more cancers and more cancer deaths than any other known agent; is a prime risk factor for heart and blood vessel disease, chronic bronchitis, and emphysema; and is a frequent cause of complications in pregnancies and of babies born prematurely, underweight, or with potentially fatal respiratory and cardiovascular problems.

Since the release of the Surgeon General's first report on smoking in 1964, the proportion of adult smokers has declined substantially, from 43% in 1965 to 30.5% in 1985. Since 1965, 37 million people have quit smoking. Although there is still much work to be done if we are to become a "smoke-free society," it is heartening to note that public health and public education efforts—such as warnings on cigarette packages and bans on broadcast advertising—have already had significant effects.

In 1835, Alexis de Tocqueville, a French visitor to America, wrote, "In America the passion for physical well-being is general." Today, as then, health and fitness are front-page items. But with the greater scientific and technological resources now available to us, we are in a far stronger position to make good health care available to everyone. And with the greater technological threats to us as we approach the 21st century, the need to do so is more urgent than ever before. Comprehensive information about basic biology, preventive medicine, medical and surgical treatments, and related ethical and public policy issues can help you arm yourself with the knowledge you need to be healthy throughout your life.

FOREWORD

Dale C. Garell, M.D.

Advances in our understanding of health and disease during the 20th century have been truly remarkable. Indeed, it could be argued that modern health care is one of the greatest accomplishments in all of human history. In the early 1900s, improvements in sanitation, water treatment, and sewage disposal reduced death rates and increased longevity. Previously untreatable illnesses can now be managed with antibiotics, immunizations, and modern surgical techniques. Discoveries in the fields of immunology, genetic diagnosis, and organ transplantation are revolutionizing the prevention and treatment of disease. Modern medicine is even making inroads against cancer and heart disease, two of the leading causes of death in the United States.

Although there is much to be proud of, medicine continues to face enormous challenges. Science has vanquished diseases such as smallpox and polio, but new killers, most notably AIDS, confront us. Moreover, we now victimize ourselves with what some have called "diseases of choice," or those brought on by drug and alcohol abuse, bad eating habits, and mismanagement of the stresses and strains of contemporary life. The very technology that is doing so much to prolong life has brought with it previously unimaginable ethical dilemmas related to issues of death and dying. The rising cost of health care is a matter of central concern to us all. And violence in the form of automobile accidents, homicide, and suicide remains the major killer of young adults.

In the past, most people were content to leave health care and medical treatment in the hands of professionals. But since the 1960s, the consumer of medical care—that is, the patient—has assumed an increasingly central role in the management of his or her own health. There has also been a new emphasis placed on prevention: People are recognizing that their own actions can help prevent many of the conditions that have caused death and disease in the past. This accounts for the growing commitment to good nutrition and regular exercise, for the fact that more and more people are choosing not to smoke, and for a new moderation in people's drinking habits.

People want to know more about themselves and their own health. They are curious about their body: its anatomy, physiology, and biochemistry. They want to keep up with rapidly evolving medical technologies and procedures. They are willing to educate themselves about common disorders and diseases so that they can be full partners in their own health care.

The ENCYCLOPEDIA OF HEALTH is designed to provide the basic knowledge that readers will need if they are to take significant responsibility for their own health. It is also meant to serve as a frame of reference for further study and exploration. The ENCYCLOPEDIA is divided into five subsections: The Healthy Body; the Life Cycle; Medical Disorders & Their Treatment; Psychological Disorders & Their Treatment; and Medical Issues. For each topic covered by the ENCYCLOPEDIA, we present the essential facts about the relevant biology; the symptoms, diagnosis, and treatment of common diseases and disorders; and ways in which you can prevent or reduce the severity of health problems when that is possible. The ENCYCLOPEDIA also projects what may lie ahead in the way of future treatment or prevention strategies.

The broad range of topics and issues covered in the ENCYCLOPEDIA reflects the fact that human health encompasses physical, psychological, social, environmental, and spiritual well-being. Just as the mind and the body are inextricably linked, so, too, is the individual an integral part of the wider world that comprises his or her family, society, and environment. To discuss health in its broadest aspect it is necessary to explore the many ways in which it is connected to such fields as law, social science, public policy, economics, and even religion. And so, the ENCYCLOPEDIA is meant to be a bridge between science, medical technology, the world at large, and you. I hope that it will inspire you to pursue in greater depth particular areas of interest and that you will take advantage of the suggestions for further reading and the lists of resources and organizations that can provide additional information.

CHAPTER 1

. . . .

THE INVENTION OF ADOLESCENCE

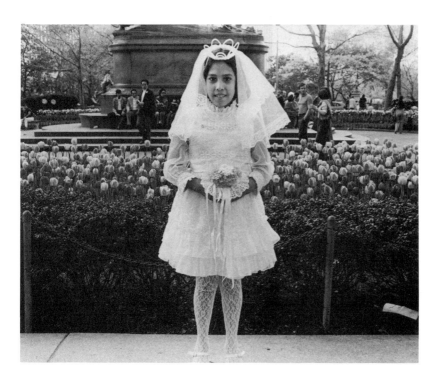

In 1909, Arnold van Gennep, a French scholar of folklore and anthropology, noted that nearly all human cultures mark certain crucial points in the life span—birth, puberty, marriage, and death—with special ceremonies or rituals. He also realized that, even in cultures separated by thousands of miles or thousands of years, many of these ceremonies and rituals contain remarkably similar elements. Van Gennep called these events "rites of passage" because they serve as a formal symbol of the individual's passage from one state of life into another. Anthropologists have continued to use this phrase, especially with regard to the ways in which societies celebrate their young people's passage from childhood to adulthood, usually around the time of puberty, or the early teenage years.

Van Gennep discovered that many rites of passage include a symbolic form of death, as if the child who is becoming an adult must shed his or her old identity, or "die" as a child, in order to be "reborn" in an adult state. One widely used symbol of this rebirth is a name change; a boy or girl will give up a childhood name at puberty and take a new, adult name.

He or she may also be isolated from society for some period of time. Among the Tukuna people of the northwestern Amazon River basin in South America, a girl undergoes a rite of passage when she has her first menstrual period. She is kept in a special small chamber inside her parents' home for up to three months. During this time, her soul is believed to wander in the under-world, or the world of spirits. At the end of this seclusion, she is "reborn" into her community, which welcomes her with a special song that compares her to a butterfly coming out of its cocoon. Like a caterpillar, she entered the chamber a child; she emerges a woman.

Rites of passage are important not just to the individual who undergoes them but to the entire society. They provide an order, a structure, that helps to bind communities. In many traditional African cultures, for example, young men belong to age sets, or groups consisting of all the males between certain ages. From childhood, members of the same age set play and receive training together. At puberty, they are banished from the community for a ritual period of seclusion, during which they live in a separate building or in the forest. Then all are circumcised or scarred in a group ceremony, after which they enter society together as men. The bonds between age-mates continue throughout their life and form part of the foundation upon which life in the community is built.

In many parts of the world, this type of one-time ceremony or event is sufficient to make any child or young person an adult in the eyes of the entire society. In the modern industrial nations of the West, however, rites of passage are less clear cut and universal. This is especially true in the United States, with its blend of many cultures and ways of life.

Instead, there are many different types of passage rites in American society. The coming-out, or debutante ball, that marks the entry into adult society of an upper-class girl; the sweet sixteen party that celebrates a girl's 16th birthday; graduation ceremonies that mark the end of high school, junior high, or even elementary school; proms and homecoming dances with their ritual election of king and queen—all of these are ways for society to acknowledge that children are becoming adults. Religious rites of passage, such as the bar and bat mitzvah for Jews and confirmation for many Christians, help young people to become members of their religious community in their own right rather than simply as their parents' children. Some rites of passage— such as a girl's first menstrual period, a boy's first shave, obtaining a driver's license, a first sexual experience, or registering to vote—are not publicly celebrated, but they are privately recognized as milestones on the road to adulthood.

Unlike a Tukuna youth, however, a young person in the industrial West today cannot cross the gap between childhood and adulthood with only one such rite of passage. A boy knows that having his bar mitzvah does not mean that he is ready to leave his parents' home, support himself, and get married; a girl knows that her sweet sixteen party is not enough to make her an adult. Individuals, families, communities, and societies continue to recognize and to celebrate the passage to adulthood with rites old and new, but the passage is no longer a single step; it is an entire stage of life, and it is called adolescence.

THE HISTORY OF ADOLESCENCE

Adolescence has not always been recognized as a distinct stage of human life, in part because prehistoric and ancient civilizations did not think that individuals developed through a number of stages. People were either children or adults, and children were regarded as small, incomplete adults, not as beings with ways of thinking and feeling that were unlike those of older people. Once children were able to support themselves, to have their own children, or to carry out some other task of adult society, they were simply considered to be adults, with adult responsibilities and privileges. Of course, it was obvious that the smaller and younger "adults" were not as strong, as experienced, or as capable as were the larger and older adults, but this was believed to be because they were smaller and younger, not because they belonged to a different stage of life development entirely.

The classical Greek and Roman civilizations, however, which existed from about 500 B.C. to about A.D. 400, did recognize a stage of life that came to be called adolescence, from the Latin verb *adolescere*, meaning "to grow up." During this time, certain young people were able to postpone some adult responsibilities while they received extended education or training in philosophy, the arts, religion, or other areas.

This adolescence, however, was not part of everybody's life; instead, it was a privilege granted by society to the children—usually the sons—of the wealthy or noble. The writings of Plato (ca. 428–347 B.C.) state that the followers of the philosopher Aristotle—as well as Plato himself—were young Greeks who belonged to this privileged class of adolescents. This class distinction was typical of ancient or medieval cultures; whenever "adolescence" did appear, it was among the elite. The great majority of young people bypassed adolescence and became adults as soon as they were old enough to work or have children.

The words *adolescence* and *adolescent* entered the English language in the 15th century. The English poet John Lydgate used "adolescence" in a poem dated 1430, and another Middle English poem, called "The Monk of Evesham," written by an unknown author around 1482, refers to "a certen adolescente a yonge man." Even then, however, adolescence meant nothing more than the third 7-year period of life, from ages 15 to 21. It was not understood to have special or distinctive qualities that made it different from childhood or adulthood in any way other than age.

As the end of the 18th century approached, social conditions in Europe and North America prepared the way for a new vision of adolescence. Cities grew; the first factories appeared. As machines began to replace workers and many adults were laid off, families began to depend on their children for additional income. But this surge in child labor had many critics. Adult workingmen's organizations resented the fact that children, who worked for lower wages, were taking away adults' jobs. Others were concerned about the very idea of youngsters laboring their childhood away in factory settings, and workers eager to get rid of their youthful competition played on this concern, always referring to it as "child labor" despite the fact that many working youths were actually in their teens. When legislation was eventually passed restricting child labor, however, legal precedent was set for recognizing "youth" as an additional stage of life encompassing ages 13 to 18 so that the same laws could restrict teenagers from working.

At the same time that adolescents were barred from the workplace, they began to spend more and more time in school. The skills required for working with more advanced equipment often dictated schooling simply as a practical means of ensuring employment. Before the growth of industry, most young people had worked at the family trade. Now, with new opportunities open to them, they stayed in school longer, and in the United States compulsory schooling laws soon made sure that this was the case. By 1900, the average American child left school at around age 14½, which would have seemed quite late a century before. The extended childhood, once the privilege of the few, was now available to many.

JEAN-JACQUES ROUSSEAU

Broad social trends prepared the soil, but it was the French philosopher and writer Jean-Jacques Rousseau (1712–78) who planted the seed of the modern concept of adolescence. In 1762, he published *Emile, or On Education*, one of the most influential books ever written about education. It is the fictional account of the upbringing of a boy named Emile, whose schooling is a model of Rousseau's theories about how to learn and teach. More important than his thoughts on education, however, was Rousseau's description of Emile's adolescence. He mentioned the physical changes of puberty, and he spoke of Emile's sexual urges, his confusion, the conflict he felt between childish and adult desires and behaviors, and his emotional turmoil.

Thus, in *Emile* adolescence was presented for the first time as a distinct stage of life and state of mind. Echoing the death-and-rebirth symbolism of traditional rites of passage, Rousseau called adolescence "a second birth," in which the child is born into the world of independent life with his or her own values and virtues.

Emile, wrote Rousseau, was like a ship. With the approach of puberty, the ship left the serene waters of childhood and entered

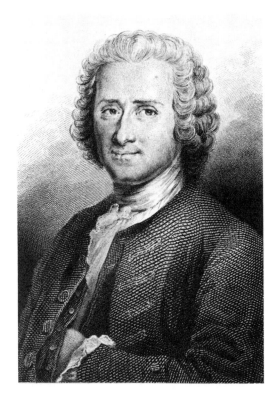

In 1762 the French philosopher Jean-Jacques Rousseau's Emile, or On Education—*one of the first books to describe adolescence—was published.*

a region of tempests and powerful waves. To avoid being capsized by these waves of emotion and passion, Emile needed to take over the steering of his ship from his childhood tutors; he had to learn to control his own passions, because self-control, as well as passion, is a part of adulthood. "Now be really free. Learn to become your own master," Rousseau told his protagonist. "Command your heart, Emile, and you will be virtuous." Like childhood, adulthood was a calm sea—but the passage between the two periods was a stormy one.

Rousseau's view of adolescence as passionate, emotional, turbulent, and sensual was seized upon by the poets and writers of the romantic period, whose work began appearing in the 1780s. The poems of William Wordsworth, Lord Byron, John Keats, and others glorified the imagination and energy of youth: Keats's "Eve of St. Agnes," for example, celebrates the life-giving passion of two young lovers, and Wordsworth, in an autobiographical poem entitled *The Prelude*, describes youth as a "golden gleam" that fades with maturity.

At about the same time, the United States was winning its independence and establishing itself as a new republic. From the start, the concept of adolescence as a vigorous, powerful, and important part of everyone's life had tremendous appeal in the United States, which was itself a young nation with a proud self-image of youthfulness, strength, and new beginnings. The next major contribution to the modern image of adolescence was made by an American.

G. STANLEY HALL

Rousseau is sometimes called the "inventor" of adolescence, but the American psychologist G. Stanley Hall (1844–1924) is regarded as the founder of the scientific study of this period of life. His two-volume study *Adolescence*, published in 1904, was the first systematic examination of adolescence as a stage in human development. Hall shared Rousseau's belief that adolescence was essentially a time of turmoil, contradictions, idealism, and emotionalism. He used the German phrase *Sturm und Drang* (storm

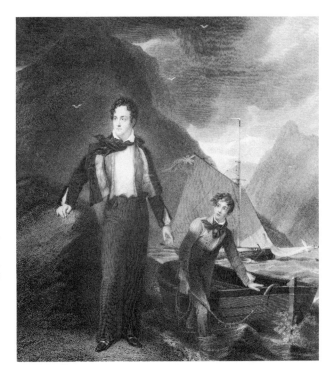

A portrait of the Romantic poet Lord Byron, whose work often celebrated the creativity and passion of youth.

and stress) to describe this quality; psychologists still use the phrase to refer to adolescent moodiness and conflict.

To Hall, as to Rousseau, adolescence meant tension and conflict between opposing forces. The adolescent feels the urgency of new sexual feelings and powers, but society's customs and rules inhibit those urges or work to prevent the adolescent from acting upon them. Similarly, the adolescent is torn between the desire to remain in the protected, dependent, comforting world of childhood and the even stronger desire to enter the independent but sometimes frightening world of adulthood. Hall noted a third source of tension in adolescent life: the conflict between individuality (the need to establish one's own identity) and conformity (the need to fit in, to belong to a group). All of these tensions contribute to the Sturm und Drang of adolescence.

Hall was influenced by Charles Darwin (1809–82), the English biologist who formulated the concept of evolution. Like Darwin, Hall regarded humankind as part of the animal world and there-

Adolescents may be torn between the desire to remain in the sheltered world of childhood and the urge to join the adult world.

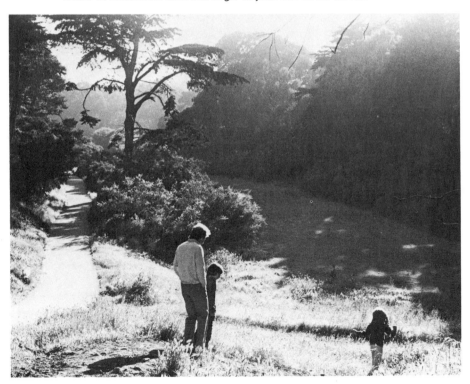

fore subject to biological laws. Hall also shared the theories of anthropologist Lewis Henry Morgan (1818–81), who believed that each stage of an individual's life recapitulates—that is, repeats or corresponds to—a period in human history.

According to Hall, infancy, when people crawl on all fours, represents the distant era when the ancestors of humans walked on all fours. Childhood represents the era of prehistoric cave dwellers. The years just before adolescence, from ages 8 to about 12, correspond to the barbaric civilizations of the ancient world. Adolescence, from ages 12 to about 25, can be compared to the origins of modern civilization in Greece and Rome, the heightened awareness of the Renaissance, and the stormy events of the 19th century. Hall believed that the 20th century would be an era of calmness, reason, moderation, restraint, and harmony—in other words, a parallel to responsible adulthood. Instead, one might consider it quite fortunate for adults that their behavior does not generally mirror the succession of wars that came to pass during the 1900s.

Contemporary psychologists have dismissed the theory of recapitulation because it cannot be scientifically tested or proved. But Hall's other achievements in the study of adolescence remain significant. He demonstrated that adolescents are different from both children and adults not simply in their level of physical development and their age but in the way they feel and think. He recognized that the special contribution of adolescence is the opportunity it offers each generation to test the values and moral beliefs of its parents and to form its own values and beliefs before confronting the full responsibilities of adulthood. Perhaps most important, he established adolescence as a subject and a life stage worthy of further study.

OTHER CULTURES, OTHER WAYS

The stormy image of adolescence that was "invented" by Rousseau received a serious challenge only a few decades after Hall made it popular. The challenge came from the science of cultural anthropology, which studies and compares the customs and social structures of various cultures. In the 1920s and 1930s, the American anthropologist Margaret Mead (1901–78) studied adolescence among some tribal peoples of Samoa, an island group in the central Pacific Ocean, and New Guinea, a large jungle island in the western Pacific. She found an almost total absence of the Sturm und Drang that Rousseau and Hall had claimed were essential to adolescence. Instead of the emotional and turbulent life stage that Rousseau and Hall had described, Mead demonstrated that, in many cultures, children move smoothly, happily, and without stress or conflict into adult roles and responsibilities. This new image of adolescence was first presented to the public in Mead's book *Coming of Age in Samoa* in 1928.

Studies by Mead and other cultural anthropologists showed that adolescence as it is experienced in the modern United States and in other Westernized, industrialized nations does not exist in all parts of the world. The biological processes of growth and development are universal; all children grow larger and, at a certain point in their growth, acquire reproductive capabilities. But not all individuals experience the same feelings about this development, and not all societies view it in the same way.

For example, a number of Asian and African cultures traditionally have had no need for prolonged training of the young, so children are encouraged to gain status by becoming adults. In these so-called continuous cultures, children typically have a fair amount of responsibility, play games mimicking adult "work," play a parental role with younger siblings, and are not discouraged from sexual experimentation at an early age.

Ruth Benedict (1887–1948), who distinguished the United States's "discontinuous" culture from this model, suggested that the existence of continuous cultures shows that adolescence as Americans define it may not be a naturally occurring stage of life at all but simply one that has appeared in many Western societies as a result of their particular conventions. In Europe and the United States, children are expected to enter the intermediate stage of adolescence and to remain in it for some time, perhaps until they have finished college or found a job that will allow them to support themselves.

Even within American culture, there are many different ways of marking adolescence. The period can be defined according to age; it is generally taken to encompass the years between 10 and 21. Alternatively, however, adolescence may be viewed primarily as a period of psychological development, occurring over a different number of years for each individual. During this time, the small, self-centered world of the child expands to include expe-

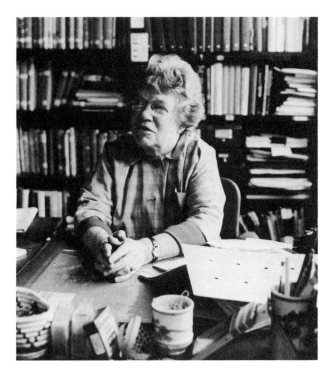

The anthropologist Margaret Mead discovered that adolescents in some less industrialized countries are able to make the transition from childhood to adulthood without the stress and conflict that their Western counterparts often endure.

riences, ideas, and feelings that will prepare him or her for life in the wider adult world.

Yet another way to view adolescence is as a period during which an individual is expected to take on certain responsibilities in the society at large. According to this definition, an adolescent is someone who is gradually moving away from childhood dependence to adulthood independence, from being part of his or her parents' family to being a recognized member of society on his or her own.

This state of having one's own standing in society is called *autonomy*, and society recognizes it in a number of ways: the right to participate in electing government representatives; the right to own property or money; and the obligation to take full legal responsibility for crimes or debts, among other ways. In cultures where adolescence exists as a prolonged state of transition, as it does in the United States, individuals who are moving toward autonomy may be granted different rights at different times. In many states, for example, a young person can stand trial as an adult for a violent crime at age 14, can quit school at age 16, and can purchase alcohol at age 21.

Perhaps the most simple definition of adolescence is a biological one, because all individuals experience the same bodily changes during their teenage years. This period of change is known as puberty; it ends when the body has developed mature reproductive capabilities. Because they happen to everyone and are the easiest changes to see and measure, these signs of physical growth are probably the most universal means of determining when someone can be considered an adolescent. Contemporary Western societies often define adolescence as a period beginning slightly before the onset of puberty and continuing for a number of years afterward; thus, puberty and adolescence do not match up as precisely parallel events. But puberty remains a key experience shared by all adolescents

It is important to remember, however, that individual boys and girls display countless variations in physical development just as they do in emotional, mental, and social development. "Normal," or "healthy," development is a very broad category. All young people move through the same stages of physical growth during adolescence, but no two individuals move through these stages at exactly the same speed. In addition, the precise end results of their adolescent growth can differ in a great number of ways, all of which are perfectly healthy, normal, and worth taking pride in.

•   •   •   •

CHAPTER 2

. . . .

PUBERTY AND
PHYSICAL
DEVELOPMENT

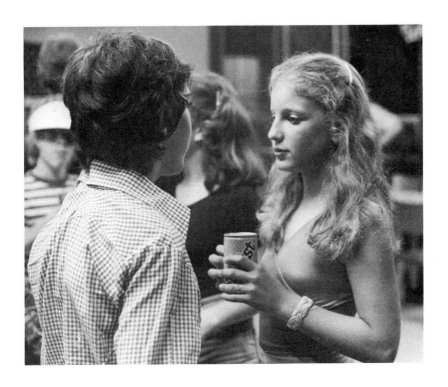

The physical changes that occur during puberty have been detailed most clearly by James M. Tanner, in his influential book *Growth at Adolescence*, published in 1962. Tanner divided the key physical changes of adolescence, such as breast development in girls, into a series of five stages that can be clearly marked and defined. These stages range from prepubescent (stage one) to adult (stage five). The initial change may occur at a later age in some individuals than in others, but Tanner's work showed that development nevertheless follows the same basic pattern.

Tanner's staging is also significant because it demonstrates how puberty occurs as a gradual process, usually spread over four to five years. Although every adolescent goes through the five stages, great differences exist in how quickly this process is completed. Different changes occur in the two sexes as well, of course, but the end results are the same for all adolescents: they achieve sexual, or reproductive, maturity and they arrive at their full adult size and strength.

In both sexes, the changes that occur during puberty are initiated by an organ called the *hypothalamus*, which lies near the middle of the brain. The hypothalamus is relatively inactive during childhood, but at the onset of puberty it begins to stimulate various glands throughout the body, including the pituitary, adrenal, and thyroid glands. These glands are all part of the endocrine system, meaning that they produce body-regulating substances called hormones. It is hormones that cause the physical changes associated with puberty.

ADOLESCENT GROWTH IN GIRLS

The commonly heard phrase "girls mature earlier than boys" may refer to emotional or social maturity in particular cases, but as a general observation about the sexes, it is based on the realities of physical growth. In general, girls do begin the process of physical development associated with adolescence at an earlier age than do boys—usually about 12 to 18 months earlier.

One major change that both boys and girls experience during puberty is a gain in both height and weight. The weight gain is less frequently discussed, and some adolescents may thus be concerned by it, but it is perfectly normal. So is the often striking "growth spurt," a period of rapid development caused primarily by a growth hormone released by the *pituitary gland*. The pituitary, an extremely important force during puberty, is located almost directly below the hypothalamus at the base of the brain.

Although girls experience the growth spurt around age 12, boys grow most rapidly around age 14. But this is a change that both sexes experience in a fairly similar way. The changes that are

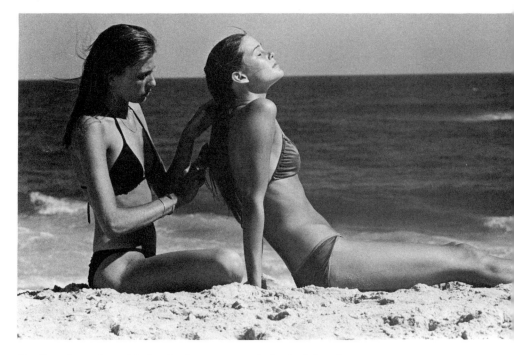

Studies show that girls begin the process of physical development at a younger age than boys.

specific to only one sex are called sexual characteristics, of which two types exist: primary and secondary. These are the physical differences that separate women from men. The differences occur because, aside from growth hormone and a few other minor hormones that are produced in significant quantities in both sexes, the hormones associated with pubertal changes differ in males and females.

Women's primary sexual characteristic is the ability to become pregnant and bear children. Female secondary sexual characteristics include pubic hair, body hair (most often under the arms and on the legs, but sometimes also in other areas, such as around the nipples), developed breasts, and hips that are usually wider than the waist. These secondary sexual characteristics begin to emerge at the same time that a girl experiences a growth spurt in height.

The increase in body hair generally takes place during early puberty. The amount of pigment in the hair also increases at this time, so that many girls between the ages of 10 and 12 find that their hair becomes darker or changes in texture. At the same time, the bone structure of a girl's pelvis begins to remold into a new shape, with a wider, higher arch between the hipbones to facilitate childbirth. And also during these early pubertal years, breast development begins.

The reason why girls develop breasts and boys do not is that breast development is primarily stimulated by two specifically female sex hormones, *estrogen* and *progesterone*. Like specifically male hormones, these are released not by the pituitary gland but by the *gonads*, or sex glands. In men, the gonads are the testes; in women, they are the ovaries. In a chain of hormonal reactions, a hormone called gonadotropin-releasing hormone (Gn-RH), secreted by the hypothalamus, triggers the release of two other hormones, luteinizing hormone (LH) and follicle-stimulating hormone (FSH). These in turn stimulate the ovaries to begin producing estrogen and progesterone.

Stimulated by these sex hormones, the process called breast budding generally occurs at around age 10 or age 11; often it is the first sign that puberty has begun. During this phase, the flat breasts of childhood become slightly elevated. The breasts continue to enlarge during the following three years or so, and the nipples generally become somewhat larger, darker, and higher than they were before. By about age 14 or 15, many girls have completed *primary breast development*—that is, their breasts have emerged and taken shape. In most adult women, the breasts will not be identical in size.

By this point, puberty is nearly over for many girls. Its midpoint occurs as the growth rate begins to decrease rapidly, usually around age 13. At this time, most girls experience the most dramatic physical change that occurs during adolescence: *menarche*, which is the beginning of monthly *menstruation*. A "period" of vaginal bleeding that usually lasts for about a week, menstruation is caused by cycles in the production of estrogen. Each month, the uterus, or womb, prepares for the possibility of pregnancy by building up its inner lining. If a woman does not become pregnant, this lining is shed, along with the unfertilized egg that was released by the ovaries. This is the discharge that is visible during menstruation.

Menarche, which is initiated by the production of estrogen,

progesterone, and several other specifically female hormones, always follows the beginning of the growth spurt, but it does not occur on a fixed timetable. Girls may begin having their periods as early as age 10 or as late as age 15 or age 16. In the United States and Western Europe today, the average age at menarche is 12.8 years, according to studies reviewed by Barbara Baker Sommer for her book *Puberty and Adolescence*, published in 1978. Health records from past years show that this average age has decreased gradually over the past century (although this trend stopped around 1970), and some doctors speculate that this decrease may have been related to improvements in both the control of disease and in the average diet.

The reproductive system. The ability to become pregnant and bear children, which occurs during adolescence, is the primary female sexual characteristic.

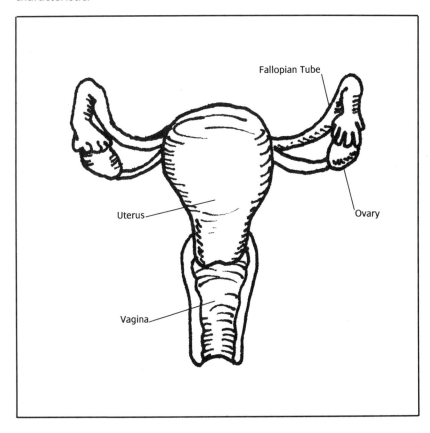

It has become widely accepted that eating habits play some role in the onset of monthly periods; very thin girls often start to menstruate considerably later than the average, whereas overweight girls frequently have an earlier menarche. Eating habits are not, however, the sole factor in determining when menarche occurs; if a girl gets her period early, this does not necessarily imply that she needs to lose weight.

Pregnancy cannot occur before menarche; thus, many people believe that a girl is able to have children as soon as she has her first menstrual period. Often, however, this is not the case. The ovaries are usually not ready to release eggs until 12 to 18 months after regular menstruation begins, so that menstruation during the earlier months is often anovulatory, or "without eggs." Not until a girl's ovaries have begun the regular production and release of eggs—a milestone in development that is not accompanied by any visible signs or changes—has she achieved reproductive maturity.

Although puberty, as it is defined, tends to end around age 14 or age 15, adolescent physical growth does not end there. Changes continue during later adolescence as well, although at a slower pace than during puberty.

During late adolescence, the menstrual cycle gradually becomes more regular, or closer to a 28-day cycle. It is not at all unusual for a girl's menstrual period to occur at irregular intervals and to vary in length during the first few years after menarche. By their twenties, however, most women can expect to have established a regular, predictable cycle of menstruation. In addition, some of the discomfort that many teenage girls experience during menstruation, such as abdominal cramping, water retention, depression or irritability, and breast tenderness, may ease as they leave their teenage years. Some girls, of course, never experience these symptoms at all. But it is important to recognize that these symptoms are extremely normal and frequently become less burdensome in later years.

Some growth in height and weight occurs after puberty, although on the average girls grow only two more inches after menarche. Many will also have experienced the full development of secondary sexual characteristics. Their voices will deepen slightly; their body hair will probably grow darker, thicker, or curlier than when it first appeared; and, in the process called *secondary breast development*, their breasts will fill out to their full adult form.

ADOLESCENT GROWTH IN BOYS

Scientists are not sure why most boys enter the process of physical development at a later age than do most girls. For boys, the growth spurt is the first sign of puberty. The male growth spurt usually begins at about age 14, as opposed to age 12 for girls. Typically, boys gain height very rapidly, sometimes shooting up six inches or so in a single year. In the first years of puberty, boys tend to add skeletal mass at a faster rate than they add muscle mass. This means that their height increases more quickly than does their weight, so that many boys in this phase of development have a lean, lanky look. This rapid increase in height, combined with growth of the hands and feet, can make an adolescent boy look and feel somewhat awkward or clumsy, but this stage of growth is both normal and temporary.

As in the female, puberty in males also brings development of the primary and secondary sexual characteristics. The male primary sexual characteristic is the ability to fertilize a woman's egg; the organs involved are the penis and the testes. Male secondary sexual characteristics include facial, pubic, and body hair and a noticeable deepening of the voice. As in girls, these sex-related changes are controlled by sex-specific hormones. In boys, the primary sex hormone is called *testosterone*; it is one of a general class of hormones known as androgens. Girls also have *androgens*, which are released by the adrenal gland and stimulate growth of typically female body hair. Because men have many more of these hormones, however, they usually have more body hair than do women.

Men's high level of testosterone is also responsible for the other male secondary sex characteristics. Stimulated by this hormone during puberty, the testes increase in size and become more prominent, and pubic hair begins to appear. Along with the increase in the boy's height comes growth of his penis. Penis growth usually starts by age 13, although it is not abnormal for this phase of development to begin a year or two later.

Just as menarche, or the onset of menstruation, signals the midpoint of puberty in girls, the midpoint of male puberty is marked by *semenarche*, or first *ejaculation*. This is the emission from the penis of the fluid known as *semen*, which is composed of sperm diluted in a bath of seminal fluid, whose purpose during sexual intercourse is simply to carry the sperm along to the female counterpart, the egg.

Usually, but not always, ejaculation of semen follows an episode of sexual stimulation or excitement. Most boys begin to experience penis erection and ejaculation by about age 12, although it is not uncommon for these experiences to begin several years earlier or later. Often the ejaculations occur at night, during sleep; these are called *nocturnal emissions*. But semenarche does not mean that a boy has become sexually mature any more than menarche means that a girl is ready to bear children. The semen of a boy's early emissions does not contain fully developed sperm. Between ages 13 and 16, the sperm mature and become capable of reproduction. When this happens, however, there is no external or visible change to show that it has occurred.

Because their growth spurt tapers off gradually rather than declining sharply like that of girls, boys experience more growth

Adolescent boys tend to increase in height extremely rapidly—as much as six inches in a single year—without gaining a substantial amount of weight.

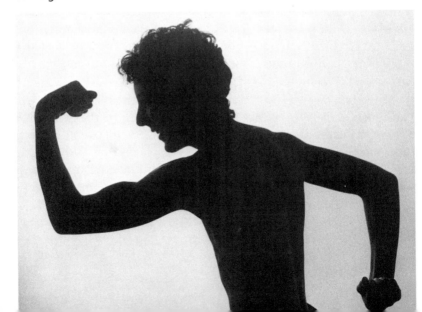

during the middle and later parts of adolescence than do girls. The postpubertal phase of physical development generally lasts several years longer for boys than for girls, ending somewhere between ages 18 and 21. Skeletal growth, or increase in height, ends at about age 17 for 50% of boys and at age 21 for an additional 33%. Boys also continue to gain muscle mass during postpuberty, as their bodies approach adult size and strength. For most boys, such growth occurs most rapidly between ages 15 and 17.

At the same time, other physical processes are under way. A boy's voice usually begins to "break," or change pitch, during early puberty. This process continues into late adolescence, and the voice becomes significantly deeper between ages 16 and 18. These years also see an increase in the amount of facial and body hair, which usually becomes somewhat darker and thicker as well. Another feature of late adolescence for many boys is the formation of an indented hairline above the forehead; the hairlines of most young boys are smooth, straight lines, but indentations, known as "widow's peaks," often appear during the late teenage years, caused by the hormones that govern the increased growth of body hair.

THE ADOLESCENT BODY

Although the changes that occur in boys' and girls' bodies during adolescence are intended to produce the same results—sexually mature adults who are capable of having children—innumerable differences exist in how quickly and to what degree each adolescent will develop during puberty. These differences are perfectly normal, yet because American culture often associates certain physical types with sexual expertise or the lack thereof, many adolescents may worry if their body's development strays from what they perceive to be "the norm."

The size of the organs associated with sex is a concern for both boys and girls. Girls are often concerned with the size of their breasts, which are the most visible signs of their developing sexuality. Large breasts are often associated with sexual activity, an association that is both unfair and quite ungrounded, because breast size is a genetically determined physical trait. Ironically, whereas some girls may thus be embarrassed by early or especially large breast development and may be teased for it, girls with smaller breasts often worry that they are lagging behind their friends. These smaller-breasted girls may have been taught that boys always prefer girls with large breasts, which is merely another myth. In fact, boys may have a very similar worry about the size of their penis because of the false link between size and sexual ability.

These kinds of generalizations are not only wrong; they are damaging to adolescents, who need to be aware that many different body types exist and that this variation is entirely healthy and normal. Few people actually fit the unrealistic standards of physical attractiveness presented by magazines and television. But because these images are so often used to define sex appeal, they have a tremendous impact on how people view their body.

Indeed, negative body image often extends beyond sexual characteristics. Adolescents of both sexes may be concerned about acne, which is another by-product of the hormonal activity associated with puberty. During the adolescent years, the skin's chemistry changes, and oil glands often become more active, causing skin disturbances such as blackheads and pimples to appear. In 1978, Robert E. Grinder published the results of studies that showed that 85% of adolescents experience some degree of acne during the preadolescent or teen years. It usually worsens in the years around puberty and tends to be more of a problem for boys than for girls, although both sexes may suffer from the condition.

Studies show, however, that adolescent girls generally worry more about their appearance than do boys of the same age. One survey of college students, published in John S. Dacey's book *Adolescents Today* in 1979, found that 75% of the males felt good about their overall looks, but only 45% of the females felt good about theirs. Part of this disparity may be explained by a 1976 survey published in *Adolescence* magazine entitled "Physical Attractiveness, Physical Effectiveness, and Self-Concept in Late Adolescence," by R. M. Lerner, J. B. Orlos, and J. R. Knapp. Most of the girls in this survey judged their looks primarily according to their sense of their social appeal, whereas the boys tended to value physical competence, or how their bodies could influence their environment, more highly. Magazines and advertisements directed at girls tend to emphasize the use of makeup, clothes, and an unrealistically thin body type as ways of attracting boyfriends; thus, it is sad but unsurprising that so many teenage girls are unable to meet the high standards of beauty that they set for themselves.

At its most devastating, this obsession with looking perfect can lead to eating disorders such as *anorexia nervosa*, in which sufferers, 90% of whom are girls, diet to the point of starvation, and *bulimia*, in which throwing up food after a meal is used as a tactic to stay thin. Although a number of other factors, such as family instability or pressure to succeed, can influence girls toward these eating disorders, studies have shown that many who suffer from these diseases first begin dieting after being teased or criticized about their weight by adults or peers.

It is important for adolescents of both sexes to recognize that overall health is much more important than being as thin as a model in a magazine. Most such models are not the ideal weight for their height but in fact are too thin, both because of the particular physical ideals of the late 20th century and because of the old saw that "the camera adds 10 pounds to your figure." Adolescents who do not plan to embark on a modeling career have the luxury of concentrating instead on how they present themselves in everyday life. Here, a nutritious diet is much more advantageous than is a drastically reduced one.

In fact, adolescence is a time of life in which good nutrition is especially important. Physical growth does not sustain itself; like any other construction process, it requires raw material. The body needs calcium for skeletal growth and protein for muscle growth. Adolescents who do not receive enough of these nutrients may not reach their full height, strength, or size. A 1969 study comparing patterns of nutrition and adolescent physical development in seven Latin American and seven Asian countries found that young people in the countries with lower average nutrition reached their growth spurt as much as two years later than did the adolescents in the countries with better nutrition. Other physical signs of puberty were also significantly delayed.

But in spite of the importance of getting enough of the right kinds of food during adolescence, many people have poorer eating habits as adolescents than they did as children. The meals children eat are usually selected, prepared, and provided by adults, but most teenagers make far more of their own food choices than do children. Because food, like clothing, is one of the areas in which young people are first able to feel some independence and control over their life, they naturally tend to choose the foods they like or those favored by their friends rather than those that are "good" for them. One health challenge adolescents face is that of combining their own tastes and their growing freedom of personal choice with a recognition of their body's nutritional needs.

•　　　•　　　•　　　•

CHAPTER 3
. . . .
CHANGES IN EMOTIONS AND THOUGHTS

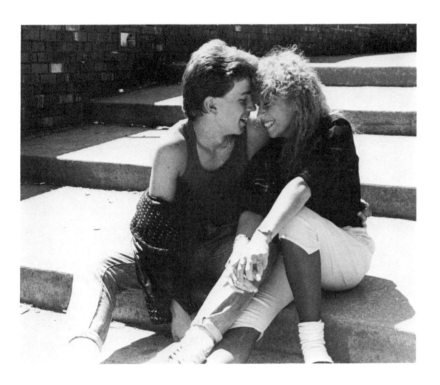

The changes that take place in the body of an adolescent boy or girl are matched by equally profound changes in how he or she thinks and feels. Unlike physical development, mental and emotional development cannot be seen or charted, although all adolescents feel their effects and show it in the things they say and do. But just as each individual develops physically at a different rate and in a slightly different way, the psychological development of adolescence is a highly individual process—and "normal" is a very broad category.

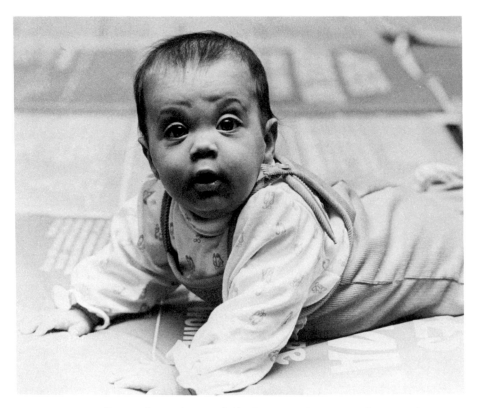

According to the Swiss psychologist Jean Piaget, an infant's understanding comprises only what he or she can readily sense.

INTELLECTUAL DEVELOPMENT

Jean Piaget (1896–1980), a Swiss psychologist, considered the growth of the intellect, or thinking mind, during the adolescent years to represent the flowering of the final, mature stage of human understanding. Piaget observed children as they passed through different levels of learning, and from these studies he created a model of cognitive, or mental, growth in which each individual passes through four stages of intellectual development on the way from infancy to maturity.

In the first three of these stages, the growing child gradually learns ways of understanding his or her environment. For the very young infant, this understanding takes place on a rudimentary level and involves only what the child can readily sense; the child has no concept of the existence of objects outside his or her own interaction with them. As the child grows older, this small, self-enclosed view of the world gradually expands to encompass the use of symbols that stand for physical objects. The child learns, for example, that a picture of a car is meant to denote an actual car and, finally, that words on a page, which look nothing like a vehicle, can also represent this physical object.

Even after this important hurdle has been cleared, however, the child still needs time to fully adapt his or her perceptions to an expanded view of the world. Specific problems in judgment remain: A five year old who sees the same amount of water poured into two different glasses—one tall and thin, one short and wide—is likely to assume that the taller glass holds more water simply because the level appears higher. Gradually, however, this child will learn that objects can have several dimensions and that a change in one may be compensated for by a change in another. With this new understanding of physical reality, a child of about eight or nine can readily classify objects or rank them according to characteristics such as amount or size.

A key, final leap occurs during Piaget's fourth stage, which he associated with the adolescent years: The young person moves

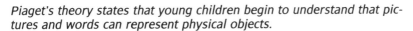

Piaget's theory states that young children begin to understand that pictures and words can represent physical objects.

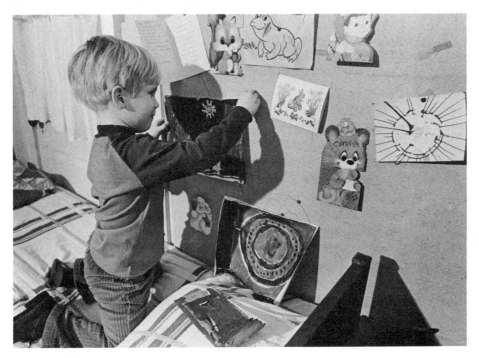

beyond an understanding of physical reality to a recognition of mental reality as well. That is, the adolescent begins to include his or her own mind in an estimation of existing realities, viewing the mind as a thing that can itself be examined and whose conclusions need not be taken for truth. Piaget called this ability evaluation, and he referred to the entire fourth stage as the achievement of *formal-operational thought.*

This phrase implies that adolescent reasoning is no longer confined to physical props; the individual is now able to form theories, to think in abstract rather than concrete terms, and to think about possibility as well as immediate reality. This last ability allows the individual to weigh possible solutions to a problem before actually trying them out; a younger child would typically go right ahead and try various solutions without considering them beforehand. The adolescent facing a problem can also take advantage of a new capability that Piaget termed *synthesis*: the ability to combine two or more sets of mental

Children in the third stage of Piaget's phases of development learn that an object's dimensions are defined not only by height but by depth and width as well.

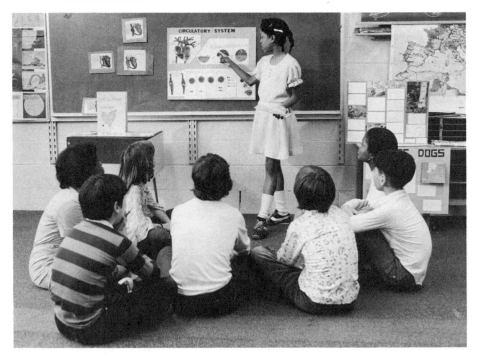

activities (logic, imagination, or factual knowledge) into a new, third pattern. Using this ability, a teenager, like an adult, is able to conceive of ideas that are both realistic and innovative.

Through their ability to understand abstract concepts, adolescents can begin to consider such subjects as death, the future, historical perspective, and personal identity—complex issues that most people spend much of their life trying to resolve for themselves. Each individual's value system, fantasies, and political beliefs, for example, are technically abstract notions, but they nevertheless play a major role in shaping a person's life.

This was Piaget's notion of the final stage of human reasoning, but other researchers have since argued that it may be problematic to assume that the ability to think abstractly is the highest goal of human thought. Perhaps, they contend, this ability is simply what is valued in American and Western European cultures rather than what is valued elsewhere. Piaget's model is thus a good example of how studies done in the United States and Western Europe need to be examined within their own particular contexts and need not necessarily be considered accurate for adolescents worldwide.

As Piaget himself stressed, many people never achieve the ability to think as described in his fourth stage. In an article published in the *Colorado Journal of Educational Research* in 1979, G. Maynard, using tasks and tests designed by Piaget himself, found that only 34% of the 18 year olds tested were capable of formal-operational thought. A year later, however, in a book called *The Emerging Adolescent: Characteristics and Educational Implications*, E. N. Brazee and P. E. Brazee found that 31% of the 12 year olds they tested were functioning according to Piaget's fourth stage. What seems clear is that intellectual development is another area in which adolescence must be viewed as a time of transition from one stage to another, a time in which the characteristics of the child and those of the adult are mingled in ways that are unique to each individual.

This process is further explained by psychologist Lawrence Kohlberg's chart of moral development. In a 1976 article entitled "Moral Stages and Moralization: The Cognitive-Developmental Approach," Kohlberg defined three types of human morality: preconventional, conventional, and postconventional. The preconventional period corresponds to childhood, when the individual is unable to see things from the point of view of others and derives

41

his or her moral standards solely from personal desires. During the conventional phase, the growing person begins to become aware of existing societal norms of "good" and "bad" and to act accordingly; this stage corresponds to the early adolescent years. Finally, Kohlberg suggested, the healthily maturing individual learns to develop morals from a postconventional perspective, in which societal norms are not taken for granted but are reflected upon in order for the individual to construct more universal moral principles. As adolescents mature, Kohlberg believed, they should begin to take a postconventional moral stance.

This stance is best accomplished when one has a strong sense of personal identity, something that Piaget also stressed. Adolescence is a time for boys and girls to achieve the self-understanding that will guide them through their adult years. In this struggle to come to terms with the self, adolescent thought often appears *egocentric*—that is, the individual mistakenly regards himself or herself as the center of everyone's attention. This does not necessarily mean that adolescents consider themselves to be especially powerful or important, although egocentrism may take this form; it often manifests itself in an opposite way, so that the adolescent feels that his or her faults or shortcomings are magnified and that everyone constantly notices them.

Two kinds of thinking are typical of adolescent egocentrism; psychologists have labeled them imaginary audience and personal fable. *Imaginary audience* refers to the belief adolescents often have that everyone is watching them, as if they were on a stage. The imaginary audience may applaud or approve of the adolescent's actions, or it may be critical or even hostile, thus increasing the adolescent's self-consciousness. A girl may walk into a party and feel that all eyes are on her, that everyone in the room is checking out her outfit and whispering about her. A boy may trip in the hallway at school and assume that everyone around him thinks he is clumsy and stupid. In fact, such feelings are in most cases quite unfounded.

Piaget suggested that these thoughts result from the adolescent's growing ability to imagine the thoughts and perceptions of other people. As they go through the process of the four stages, Piaget believed, children gradually learn that a world exists outside the self and that other people think and feel too. When adolescents realize this, they may become concerned that others are thinking about them. As adolescents interact more and more with their peers and with adults outside the family, they learn to distinguish valid perceptions from imaginary audience sensations.

A second kind of egocentric thinking that is common during adolescence is the *personal fable*: a myth or fallacy that adolescents wish to believe about themselves. Using this technique, young people can imagine themselves doing things they might never attempt in reality. Personal fables can thus provide a healthy means of exploring one's identity. Many personal fables have their origins in preadolescent daydreaming, when, for example, a child may fantasize that he or she is really the child of wealthy or royal parents or has a secret identity as a spy or superhero.

An adolescent personal fable may be a way for a young person to believe that he or she is unique, special, and different from everybody else—and establishing this belief is a natural and necessary part of the process of building a mature identity. Thus, personal fables can play an important role in fostering imagination, creativity, self-confidence, and a strong sense of self.

On the negative side, studies have shown that sometimes personal fable thinking is exaggerated by adolescents who appear to believe that they are invulnerable to the ordinary laws of nature and rules of everyday life. An all-too-common example of this misconception is the young couple who engage in intercourse, knowing full well the risk of pregnancy but not taking precautions. The couple may have convinced themselves that *they* are not vulnerable to the same risk other couples are. This kind of distorted thinking has contributed to (but is by no means the sole cause of) the ever-growing number of teenage pregnancies, including many that result from first intercourse.

Normally, this kind of negative personal fable thinking diminishes as the individual develops more intimate relationships and realizes that he or she is not so different from everyone else after all; in fact, he or she may have feelings in common with others that are assumed to be the strangest of individual problems or fears. It is only when personal fables become obsessive, interfere with relationships with other people, or begin to conflict in serious ways with what the adolescent knows to be true that they can block normal development rather than enhance it. For most people, daydreams and fantasies continue throughout adulthood and are generally regarded by psychologists as being perfectly healthy and normal as long as the daydreamer does not confuse them with reality.

In addition to being egocentric in the ways mentioned above, adolescent thought is often idealistic, critical of others (especially adults), uncompromising, and given to absolutes—adolescents often see things as black or white rather than in shades of gray. Like egocentrism, these features of adolescent thought are the result of the young person's need to build an independent identity. One way to do this is to establish strong values and opinions of one's own and to express them. For many young people, this means rebelling against their parents' ideas and values.

Piaget considered adolescents' questioning of the wisdom handed down by their elders to be healthy, on the whole; it keeps society flexible, creative, and progressive. Often during the course of American history, such as during the political upheavals of the 1960s, it has been young people who have led the way in calling for social change and who in doing so have shaped the way society views things today.

Of course, a balance is important between incessantly pushing for one's own views and respecting the views of other people, from parents to peers. Like all other skills, mental processes such as identifying personal values, organizing logical arguments, and creating theories about the world require practice and refinement. With time, most adolescent thinkers acquire the skills of compromise, give-and-take, and accommodating other people's beliefs.

EMOTIONAL DEVELOPMENT

Just as Piaget's model of cognitive growth offers a useful framework for examining intellectual development during adolescence, Erik Erikson's model of psychosocial development (the development of a person's psychological well-being and social interaction) provides a way to understand the emotional side of adolescent growth. Erikson (b. 1902) is a Danish-American psychoanalyst who has studied and practiced in the United States for many years. In his study of development, he identified eight stages through which each person passes between birth and death. In each stage, the individual must resolve a conflict between two opposing forces, one that encourages healthy development and another that tends to stifle or distort personal growth.

Unlike Piaget's model of four stages for intellectual development, where adolescence marked the final phase of human understanding, Erikson's series of conflicts assumes a lifelong process, in which adolescence is simply one step in a continuing series. During childhood, the emotionally healthy child achieves the correct goal of each conflict by being given plenty of support and acknowledgment, whereas a child who is punished or neglected might follow the opposite path.

Erikson's eight stages are as follows:

1. *Trust vs. Mistrust.* During infancy, the healthy child raised by loving parents learns to feel secure by trusting others.

2. *Autonomy vs. Shame and Doubt.* Through his or her parents' approach to toilet training, the toddler either learns to be confidently independent or, if chastised, remains ashamed and self-doubting.

3. *Initiative vs. Guilt.* Healthy preschool children learn self-motivation through adult encouragement and support; if punished or neglected, children at this age may feel guilty or timid.

4. *Industry vs. Inferiority.* The elementary school child should learn, through work and social interaction, that he or she has something worthwhile to offer. If not sufficiently encouraged, a child at this age may feel ineffective or inferior.

5. *Identity vs. Role Confusion.* This is the conflict that faces adolescents. It will be discussed below.

6. *Intimacy vs. Isolation.* Young adults attempt to merge their identity with that of others in intimate relationships rather than face the world alone.

7. *Generativity vs. Stagnation.* Adults feel fulfilled through a sense of generativity, of contributing something to the world. If this is not accomplished, they may feel stagnant, or immobile.

8. *Ego Integrity vs. Despair.* In old age, the person looks back on his or her life, and if it seems whole and satisfying, the product of an integrated sense of self, he or she accepts the aging process. If not, the individual may feel despair.

Thus, the adolescent phase of Erikson's model is of particular importance; if a young person does not establish a coherent identity, Erikson believed, he or she will not be prepared to face all the subsequent conflicts of life. It was Erikson who coined the phrase *identity crisis* to refer to the profound disturbance that many young people feel as they begin to separate from their parents and family. He perceived that this process can produce a sense of alienation—that is, of being distanced from both oneself and from society. Learning to cope with this feeling of alienation, Erikson felt, is a normal part of the challenge of growing up.

Young people also face the stress of new peer relationships, changing family relationships, puberty and an emerging sexual identity, career choices, and the broader issues of the values and beliefs that will shape the adolescent's later life. Adolescents who are able to confront these expanded possibilities and integrate them into a unified, complete ego, or sense of self, will move on to Erikson's next stages; those who fail to understand and accept their new role in society may face role confusion, a state of uncertainty about the self that can prevent healthy psychological growth. This same uncertainty might result if a young person chooses too often to postpone or avoid dealing with conflicts.

It is ironic that just when young people's intellectual horizons are expanding and they begin to envision potential futures, they also feel increasing pressure to narrow those horizons by making choices. A 17 year old may be excited about applying to many different colleges but will often feel pressured by school counselors and parents to make "the right decision" when planning a future career. A high school junior might enjoy flirting with various people but could worry that this freedom might translate into being thought of as sleazy or immature.

Like Piaget's four stages, Erikson's eight conflicts have been criticized by some modern researchers, who question the universality of his approach. Erikson's model defines a healthy identity as one based on individuality, achievement, and independence—values that may not always be appropriate in social situations. Certainly, it is not always appropriate to strive only to better one's own position rather than to cooperate with others.

In addition, Esther Sales, in a 1978 study called "Women's Adult Development," and Judith Gallatin, in her 1975 book *Adolescence and Individuality*, have pointed out that in American society it is primarily men who are taught to value individual achievement above all else, whereas women are often encouraged to value cooperation and relating to others instead. Many women, Sales contended, deal with questions of intimacy, which compose the core of Erikson's next stage, before they resolve issues of their own identity. This is probably a result of the emphasis that society has traditionally placed on women to get married and have children, whereas men are more frequently expected to go out and "make a name for themselves" in a job or career.

TIMES OF STRESS

Part of what can make social interaction difficult for adolescents is the emotional stress that has typically been associated with the teenage years. Adolescent stresses cover a broad spectrum, from the arguments with parents, siblings, and friends that are part of almost everyone's life to severe traumas such as sexual abuse, the death of a parent, or an unplanned pregnancy. For the most part, however, adolescent stress is simply the result of the high intensity of emotions during the teenage years.

A number of factors combine to make many individuals' emotions stronger and more changeable during adolescence than

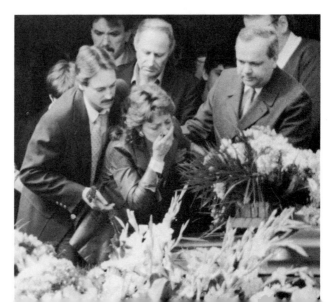

A mother mourns her teenage son, who committed suicide. Irving Weiner, an American psychologist, has theorized that most teenagers who attempt suicide are reacting to a troubled family situation in the only way they can imagine.

during any other time of life. Among these factors are changes in mental abilities, physical changes such as hormone production and sexual development, and life changes such as starting high school or beginning to separate emotionally from one's parents. The effect of all these factors on someone who is physically, mentally, and socially changing from a child to an adult can be quite confusing—both to the adolescent and to his or her family members, friends, and teachers.

Perhaps the most noteworthy feature of adolescent emotions is their unpredictability. A teenager may laugh hysterically, cry fiercely, and brood solemnly, all in the space of an hour or two and all with complete sincerity. Because adolescents' moods and feelings fluctuate from one extreme to another so quickly, adults may make the mistake of not taking them seriously or perhaps even ridiculing them. Such reactions not only reveal a misunderstanding of the nature of adolescent feelings, but they can also cause the young person to become even more excessively emotional as a form of rebellion or to stifle his or her emotions in order to avoid further ridicule or punishment. Neither course will foster healthy emotional growth.

Just as adults tend to belittle the range of adolescent emotions, many adults do not take teenagers' negative feelings seriously, which in a particularly extreme case might mean ignoring the warning signs of a suicide attempt. Teenage suicide is a serious problem in the United States today, but some adults feel that many adolescents who attempt suicide are not serious about killing themselves. Teenagers are just overreacting as usual, they contend, and are simply using a dramatic way to get attention. This theory is half right, according to psychologist Irving Weiner in his 1980 article "Psychopathology in Adolescence"; he maintained that some, although not all, teenage suicide attempts are indeed a cry for help rather than a genuine attempt to die. But it is wrong to label such actions the result of immaturity or hysteria. Most often, Weiner said, teenagers who attempt suicide are reacting to a troubled family situation in the only way that they can imagine. To help them, one must take their pain seriously and not trivialize it as the act of an immature child.

The best approach, however, is to recognize the feelings that lead to such a desperate act before such an act actually occurs. Teenagers and adults alike should learn to be aware of the particular changes in behavior that psychologists caution may point to a suicidal attitude. Unfortunately, this can be especially difficult during the adolescent years, when exaggerated emotional responses are considered normal. Most adolescents cry, argue, sulk, demonstrate affection, and laugh more than adults do. They tend to reveal their emotions through their behavior to a greater extent than do many adults, who may have trained themselves to suppress or conceal their feelings. This restraint is typical of what is expected of adults in our culture, although it is not necessarily true worldwide. In the United States, being grown up often means not showing when one is hurt or excited, because to reveal emotion may appear immature, the act of someone lacking in self-control. It is debatable, however, whether this is in fact any healthier or more "mature" than the adolescent tendency to show emotions to their fullest extent.

Emotions that adolescents tend to find most troubling include the following:

1. Fear and anxiety, often centering around the dread of appearing foolish or unattractive to others.

2. Guilt, which can arise when a behavior conflicts with values, as when someone who places a positive value on honesty finds him- or herself cheating or lying.

3. Grief, a sense of loss or deep disappointment that, if it can be expressed or shared in a supportive environment, often results in personal growth.

4. Shyness, which is usually the result of a home environment in which the adolescent is not encouraged to express him- or herself and is not rewarded for taking chances. Shyness is often best overcome through experience with group activities such as clubs, religious organizations, and classes.

5. Anger, the most powerful emotion most people experience and the one with which they often feel the least comfortable, but one that adolescents must learn to express safely and appropriately.

Several methods, which psychologists call coping strategies, exist for dealing with these feelings in a mature way. Certain of these approaches lend themselves better to certain feelings, but in time healthy adolescents will learn which work best for their particular needs. Coping strategies include the following:

1. Humor, or finding what is funny in a painful experience.

2. Self-expression, or finding someone—a parent, relative, friend, teacher, therapist, or religious counselor, for example—to whom emotions can be honestly expressed and who will respond with respect and understanding.

3. Escape, which may be harmful if overused, can offer much-needed relief from stress and may be appropriate if one feels that a situation that has been blown out of proportion might be helped by some cooling-off time. Some common escapes include watching television or daydreaming in order to avoid thinking about something unpleasant or withdrawing to a private place to avoid interaction and conflict.

4. Reflection, or self-examination, meaning analyzing one's own feelings and behavior, looking for other courses of action to follow next time, or trying to understand others' hurtful behavior.

Over time, such coping strategies can teach the adolescent to understand, control, and respect his or her feelings as well as the feelings of others. A young person who deals with his or her own emotions efficiently will do better in interactions with other people; it is this logic that Erikson followed when he argued that in order to achieve intimate relationships with others, a person must first develop a coherent sense of self.

•   •   •   •

CHAPTER 4

RELATIONSHIPS AND IDENTITY

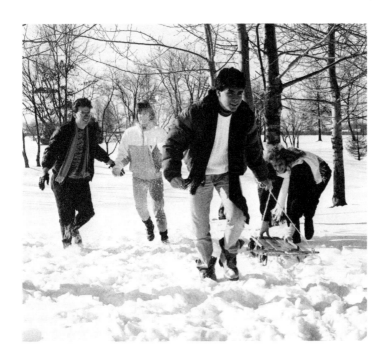

No man is an island," wrote the English poet John Donne in 1624. One of the meanings of this frequently quoted statement is that each individual life is connected to others—to what Donne called "the continent" of all humankind. Today, scientists called ethologists, who study the behavior of many species of animals (and often arrive at conclusions that lead to a greater understanding of the human animal), have divided the animal kingdom into two broad groups of species: the solitary and the gregarious. *Gregarious species* are those whose members typi-

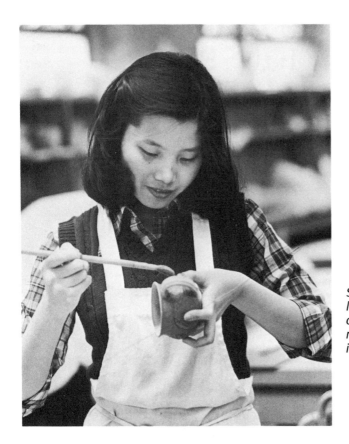

Some teenagers depend less than others on social interactions and more on individual activities such as hobbies.

cally band together in some way to form social groups. Human beings are a gregarious species.

A human being very rarely—perhaps never—exists in true isolation from other people. Babies need other people around simply to fulfill basic needs, but the need for human contact goes beyond physical survival. People require interaction with others for healthy development and for the fulfillment of their intellectual and emotional potential.

The amount and kind of interaction, however, can vary widely from person to person. For example, one teenager may feel lonely and unhappy unless he or she spends several hours with three or four close friends almost every day; another may be perfectly content to spend more free time alone pursuing a hobby or an interest and to see friends only at school or on occasional weekends.

Whatever type and degree of social contact people choose for themselves, each person must discover *how* to interact with others. Psychologists call that process of discovery *socialization*: the method by which individuals adapt to society. It is particularly important during adolescence, when young people are preparing to fill a place of their own in the world.

Socialization involves teaching and learning. Members of society, such as parents, teachers, clergy, and popular heroes, teach the values, customs, and normal behaviors of their culture, sometimes by direct teaching and sometimes simply by displaying them. Young people learn by listening to and watching others; eventually they must weigh and evaluate what they have observed and decide what to keep, what to change, and what to reject.

A very young infant begins this process by observing the adults around him or her, particularly the mother, father, or primary care giver. In order to be liked by these people, the child tries to be like them by unconsciously or instinctively imitating such acts as smiling, talking, and hugging. This same process continues in a more conscious form as the child goes through elementary school, where his or her environment expands and more people

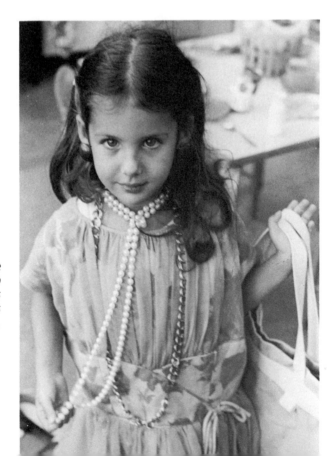

Young children begin the process of growing up by imitating the dress and behavior of adults around them.

provide clues about how to act. The child wants to do and say things that will be accepted as normal and appropriate, so he or she experiments with behavior and attitudes adopted from many different models, from parents to peers to characters in movies or on television.

As the child matures, he or she usually begins to make more thoughtful and careful selections of models to follow. Adolescents typically become concerned with concepts of right and wrong and about how their own actions will be judged by family members, friends, teachers, and others. Behavior is influenced more and more by *reinforcement* and *punishment*. If the adolescent perceives approval for his or her behavior, he or she is more likely to act that way again. But if the behavior causes the young person to feel anxious, guilty, or ashamed around others because he or she worries that they would not approve, the behavior is less likely to be repeated.

Whether behavior is reinforced or punished depends to a great extent upon whose opinion the adolescent values most. A teenager who cheats in order to pass a test in school, for example, may be applauded by some fellow students and reprimanded by teachers and other students. If the approval of the first group is more valuable to the teenager than that of the second group, the behavior will be reinforced, and the student will be more likely to cheat again on the next exam.

This particular example reflects a typical struggle for the adolescent who is trying to make decisions based on social relationships. Conflicts often arise when adults, such as teachers or parents, want the adolescent to conform to what is traditionally expected or considered "right." The adolescent's peers, however, may be judging their friend by different rules, expecting that he or she will do what is most fun for the crowd. Time and time again, a young person must decide between these two alternatives, and the decision is rarely an easy one. Family relationships shape a person's life from his or her earliest days of existence; these ties are not easy ones to ignore or cast aside.

THE ADOLESCENT AND THE FAMILY

The normal course of growth and development turns a dependent child, whose needs are filled by care givers within the family, into an independent adult, able to take care of him- or herself—

and eventually, perhaps, to care for the next generation. For this change to take place, the child must first undergo two processes; these are called individuation and separation.

Individuation takes place in infancy and early childhood, when the child realizes that he or she has an individual identity and starts to think, feel, and act on his or her own while remaining within the protective framework of the family, which may include neighbors and close family friends. *Separation* usually begins during the preadolescent years and continues throughout adolescence. The term refers to the slow, sometimes painful task of separating from the family in order to prepare for autonomy and adult responsibilities such as work and marriage. Separation is one of the most crucial challenges adolescents face; it is a process that is generally not completed until early adulthood.

Achieving emotional independence from parents does not mean that their love, approval, and emotional support will not continue to play an important part in the adolescent's life. It simply means that the need for emotional support from the parents will eventually give way to the need to be self-reliant and self-directed.

Quite often, adolescents who are going through the process of separation become critical of their home and family members; it is common in the United States for teenagers to spend more and more time away from home as they get older. And yet, because of the natural egocentricity or self-centeredness of adolescent thought, many young people forget that their parents are emotional beings, too. Quite often, a young person interprets his or her parents' opposition to new friends and new behaviors as unnecessarily harsh, when in fact the parents may be feeling hurt or rejected by their adolescent's growing interest in people outside the family. Indeed, a 1975 study by Richard M. Lerner, "Showdown at Generation Gap," showed that adolescents tend to overestimate the number of major differences between themselves and their parents, whereas parents tend to underestimate such differences. This discrepancy may be caused in part because teenagers see themselves as changing into newly independent, adult individuals, whereas their parents still look at them and see them as their little children.

Yet even young people themselves may feel an inner conflict at times between the desire for independence and the desire to remain in the comfortable, emotionally secure world of childhood dependency. At times all adolescents feel the urge to withdraw from the new experiences and sensations they are encountering; they also feel occasional pangs of loss or nostalgia as their relationship with their parents begins to change.

This ambivalence, or sensation of having opposing feelings at the same time, contributes to the emotional ups and downs of the adolescent years. A typical example of the adolescent mix of adult and childish behaviors is the 13 year old who decides that he wants to go to the movies on Saturday night with friends rather than with his family. He has chosen a more adult behavior—and yet he may cry, sulk, or otherwise demonstrate his anger in a less-than-adult fashion if denied permission to go.

Parents who see their teenage children "growing away" from the family-centered life of earlier years may not realize or wish to admit that this movement is a natural part of growing up. Such parents, perhaps fearing that their adolescents are too rebellious, may become unusually strict or authoritarian. Such attitudes will probably not make the adolescent passage any smoother for either the parents or their children. Other parents may feel that their adolescents are rejecting them and their values and may withdraw emotionally from their children, closing off avenues of communication and sharing that could help to keep the parent-adolescent relationship healthy.

What these parents may not realize is that conflict between the generations is an extremely normal and even healthy part of adolescence. A 1973 study by J. D. Schvanevedlt, published in *Adolescence* magazine, found that most American adolescents tend to clash with their parents over very similar issues. In the group that Schvanevedlt studied, these issues included personal appearance, curfew hours, the use of a car or money, chores or homework, and permission to date. Another researcher, Arlene Skolnick of the University of California at Berkeley, made a more startling discovery, reported in her 1978 book *The Intimate Environment: Exploring Marriage and Family.* Many of the most mature, creative adults whom she studied had had a particularly difficult youth.

Many adolescents experience some "storm and stress" within the family, but this usually dies down as they come to terms with

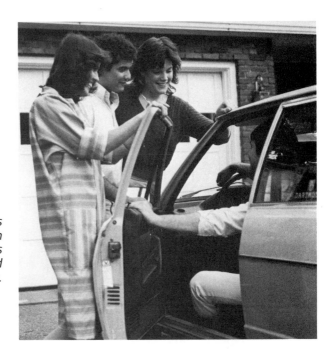

Use of the family car is one of the most common sources of arguments between adolescents and their parents.

themselves as adults. *Extremely* rebellious behavior is much less common, though many people mistakenly consider it to be typical of adolescence. In a 1975 study by J. O. Balswick and C. Macrides, published in *Adolescence* magazine, only about one-fifth of the college students surveyed described their early adolescent years as "very" or "extremely" rebellious.

When serious rebellion does occur, as when teenagers continually ignore the rules that their parents have set for them, studies have shown that parental attitudes play a major role. Either extremely restrictive or, conversely, extremely permissive attitudes on the part of parents may lead adolescents to engage in "problem" behavior, such as the use of hard drugs. An unhappy family situation is also likely to make a teenager engage in rebellious activities because he or she feels alienated from the home.

The family's economic situation may be yet another factor in how parental attitudes affect adolescent behavior. A 1975 study by Russell Curtis, published in the journal *Adolescence*, found that teenagers from middle-class homes were more likely to hold their parents' opinions in high regard, whereas adolescents from lower-class homes, who often saw their parents as incompetent or lacking in the resources necessary to conduct their life, were less likely to trust their parents' judgment and thus less likely to obey their rules.

Another study, conducted by D. B. Kandel and published in the *Journal of Personality and Social Psychology* in 1978, showed that if adolescents do turn to their parents for advice, it is usually about larger life issues, such as how to prepare for the future, whereas interactions with friends are more likely to guide teenagers' daily decisions and behavior. Although most children have friends, it is not until preadolescence that friendships and other relationships with peers become as important as relationships within the family in determining an individual's sense of self-worth and identity. In part, this new reliance on friends reflects that adolescents, eager to explore the new responsibilities open to them, can exert some authority in choosing friends, whereas few have a say in the composition of their family.

In some cases, the beliefs and behaviors of a young person's peers mirror those of his or her family; this is often the case in close-knit communities with a high degree of shared social and cultural background, as in areas of Utah where members of the Mormon faith—which forbids such activities as smoking and drinking—predominate. In such situations, the values an adolescent shares with other teenagers will probably echo, or reinforce, those of the parents.

Often, however, young people become interested in behaviors that differ from their parents' values or even that directly contradict them. This may be the result of a teenager encountering adolescents from other cultural, social, religious, racial, or economic backgrounds, often with values and habits different from those of his or her family. But one study by John Janeway Conger, described in his 1975 book *Contemporary Issues in Adolescent Development*, found that the majority of adolescents have friends from a background similar to their own, who have families of comparable income, are of the same ethnic makeup, and live in the same neighborhood. Thus, it is probably basic generational differences that spark most parent-teenager value conflicts.

In the end, disagreements between the generations may cause the adolescent to form a value system that diverges radically from that of his or her family, or he or she may decide that such a divergence is not necessary or desirable. The process of making such a decision is known as *value synthesis*. As a result of value synthesis, adolescents arrive at a set of beliefs by considering the behavior of all the people around them: parents, teachers, religious leaders, and friends. For most adolescents, exposure to people outside the family is a necessary part of value synthesis. And the primary form such exposure takes is relationships with other adolescents.

PEER GROUPS AND FRIENDSHIP

Nearly all adolescents belong to some sort of peer group, an association of friends with whom they identify themselves. During preadolescence, most friendship groups—variously called cliques, crowds, and gangs—consist of youngsters of the same sex. By the time these boys and girls reach age 14 or age 15, these same-sex peer groups will probably have begun to merge into larger, more loosely defined mixed-sex groups whose members then begin to date one another in one-on-one relationships.

Teenagers feel a powerful desire to affiliate—that is, to be associated with a group—for at least three reasons. First, the process of growing up inevitably causes a certain amount of separation from the family, and although teenagers generally welcome this autonomy, they also miss the sense of closeness and belonging that they experienced as younger children in the family. Belonging to a peer group fills the need for acceptance and closeness. Second, teenagers are struggling to establish their own identity. Peer groups offer adolescents the opportunity to experiment with a variety of values, habits, and customs that may become part of that identity. Third, peer groups are a way for adolescents to approach romantic or sexual attachments. Most adolescents take part in group outings or activities before they begin dating one-on-one.

Belonging to a group can have many positive effects. The group bolsters the adolescent's sense of self-esteem. It gives the adolescent an arena in which to practice interpersonal skills, such as communication, cooperation, and compromise, that will be important in the workplace and in adult relationships. But being part of a group has negative aspects, too, that adolescents should recognize.

For one thing, exclusion from a desired group can be painful indeed; although belonging to the "in crowd" is often a major

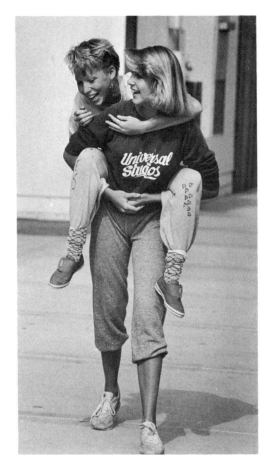

Teenage girls often have one close friend with whom they identify and empathize.

boost to one's self-esteem, few experiences in adolescence are as unpleasant as being left out of the clique one wants to join. And acceptance in a group can also be damaging; for example, the group may encourage behavior that is destructive or contrary to one's own values, or membership in the clique may begin to take precedence over all other forms of growth and self-expression, such as studying, meeting new people, or sports and hobbies.

Most adolescents must continually examine their relationship with their peer group to be sure that they are benefiting from their friendships and not being limited by them. Just as establishing oneself within a peer group is often a big step toward forming an adult identity, there may be times when an adolescent will need to leave a group in order to take the next step forward. Indeed, most adolescent peer groups have fluid boundaries, so that their membership shifts and changes often. Many adolescents belong to several different peer groups over the course of their junior high and high school years, each important in its own time.

Although belonging to a peer group is a significant part of growing up for most people, preadolescents and adolescents generally experience more intimate friendships as well. Some psychologists believe, however, that boys and girls tend to experience friendship somewhat differently. In her 1985 book *Just Friends: The Role of Friendship in Our Lives*, psychologist Lillian Rubin pointed out that teenage girls are likely to have "best friends" (usually only one friend at a time fills this role, although who the best friend is may change periodically); teenage boys, on the other hand, are somewhat more likely to identify with a small group of close friends.

Male adolescents tend to center their social interactions around group activities, such as sports.

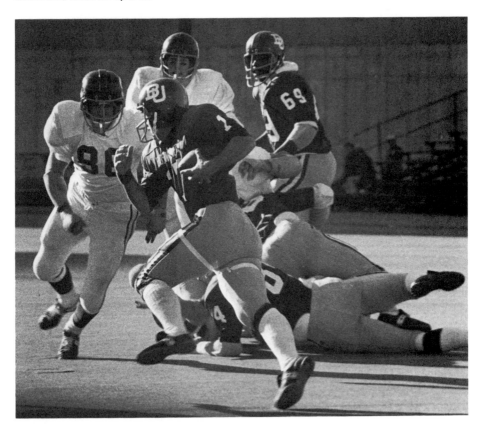

Rubin concluded that, in general, men and women have different friendship styles that may have their roots in childhood and adolescence. Men, she claimed, often list more friends than do women, but women's friendships tend to be more intimate. Men's interactions with friends are often organized around specific activities, such as work or sports, whereas woman friends may spend a higher portion of time talking, sharing their experiences and feelings. To some extent, Rubin claimed, the difference in friendship style can be seen in adolescent friendships.

Gender differences have also been noted in the way that the two sexes make moral judgments. Psychologist Carol Gilligan, in her book *In a Different Voice*, suggested that women's moral decisions tend to be based more on empathy, or identification with the feelings of other people, than on abstract concepts of right and wrong. But the women Gilligan studied often seemed to have difficulty making moral judgments at all; they appeared to feel uncomfortable about their right to do so. These differences seem consistent with Rubin's findings about gender differences in friendship, in that girls' more intimate relationships may teach them to depend more on the opinions of other people.

Many psychologists believe, however, that these differences are primarily, if not solely, the result of socialization, or the different ways in which boys and girls are taught to behave. The current social trend toward ending sex-role stereotypes may well mean that these differences, along with other differences in behavior between the sexes, will be modified in the next generation of boys and girls.

•　　　•　　　•　　　•

CHAPTER 5

TRYING OUT
ADULT
BEHAVIORS

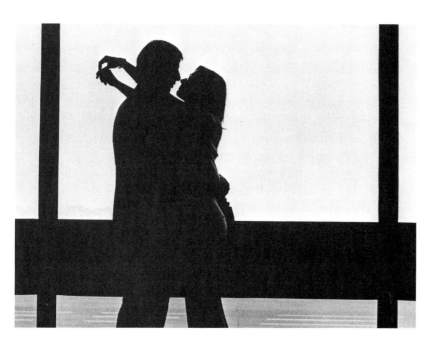

From the first rush of hormones at the onset of puberty, nearly all adolescents become interested in sexual matters. Aside from dealing with physical development, which was discussed in Chapter 3, adolescents face the challenges of becoming comfortable with their new sexual identity and of interacting with each other on a romantic level.

Still, although most people begin to think about romance and sexuality during the early years of puberty, neither boys nor girls are likely to move from preadolescence directly into confident

63

dating. Instead, young people of both sexes tend to fantasize about romantic encounters and attachments, often with public figures such as rock stars or models. The unattainability of famous people is actually advantageous here; young adolescents are free to imagine romantic scenarios precisely as they choose, leaving aside for the moment the more complex questions raised by serious involvement with another person.

The next step, however, generally strikes closer to home. It is usually a crush on, or passionate infatuation with, someone who is more of a part of the young person's own world, such as a teacher or a peer from school. In many cases, the infatuated adolescent and the object of his or her crush never meet face-to-face. But the crush serves its purpose, allowing the adolescent to imagine him- or herself in social or intimate situations with a romantic partner who is a part of his or her everyday life.

Such fantasies and crushes are perfectly normal and often continue beyond adolescence into adulthood. They are a problem only in the rare instances in which they lead the adolescent into inappropriate behavior or when they become so important that they cause teenagers to lose sight of reality and miss out on opportunities for more likely interactions.

During the high school years, many adolescents do get romantically involved with a peer. Many people have their first experience of falling in love during adolescence. This, too, is a normal part of growing up. But even though feelings of love, attachment, and desire can be extremely powerful during the adolescent years, very few teenage relationships, even the most intense, are lasting ones.

Adolescent dating can be a wonderful experience or a very painful one. It is more often the latter when one's expectations do not match up with reality. This is not uncommon, given the images teenagers are shown by the media, in which young heroes and heroines have many different romances, seemingly on a weekly basis. In real life, this situation is hardly the norm. Yet many teenagers may feel pressure to date even when they are not especially interested in anyone or when they feel unready to enter into a romance.

It is up to each adolescent to recognize when he or she is truly ready to enter into a romantic relationship with another person.

When this time comes, both people will benefit most if they judge the relationship on its own terms rather than on any expectations they may have regarding what romance is "supposed" to be all about. Each relationship is different; people express affection in different ways, and some people need a great deal more time than do others before they can open up to another person in an intimate fashion. Many adolescents find that the best kind of romantic partner is a friend first—someone from whom they can expect the same respect one would expect from a nonromantic friend. When trust and understanding give way to game playing and manipulation, it is often a sign that the relationship has become unhealthy.

Some adolescents may feel left out of "the dating game" because they feel attracted not to members of the opposite sex but to same-sex friends. Many people feel such attractions at one time or another, but only some of these people will turn out to be homosexual, meaning that they will have adult intimate relationships with members of their own sex. Most young people will gradually become aware of whether these feelings set a pattern for all of their romantic attractions. Because of all the negative associations that Western society has attached to homosexuality, admitting this to oneself can be difficult. Attitudes are gradually changing, however, and young people who question their sexual identity in this way should realize that many adults have come to the same realization and have successful, happy, romantic homosexual relationships.

Another issue that is often particularly difficult for adolescents is the question of whether or not to engage in sexual intercourse. Beliefs differ on whether sex before marriage is ever appropriate, but nevertheless an extensive 1981 survey of American teenagers, by Jane Norman and Myron W. Harris, found that 44% of all U.S. adolescents from ages 13 to 18 had had sexual intercourse. The rate was significantly higher for boys, suggesting the continued existence in the United States of the "double standard," or the traditional belief that it is more acceptable for boys to engage in sexual activity than it is for girls to do so. (It is also important to note that because of the double standard, boys are probably more likely to admit to having had sex than are women.) The persistence of this unfortunate stereotype has negative consequences for both sexes. On the one hand, many boys who are told that having sex at a young age is not only appropriate but is in fact a sign of manliness will engage in sexual relations without considering whether they are truly ready to do so. On the other hand, many girls who feel strong sexual attractions may feel guilty or worried about having these feelings because American culture has traditionally labeled girls who have sex "loose" or immoral.

These differing pressures on the two sexes are further demonstrated by studies showing that more than half of teenage boys discuss with others, within a month, their first act of sexual intercourse, whereas few girls do so. In fact, a full 40% of girls express that they wish they had waited longer, and many claim to have felt fear or anxiousness during the experience. It is significant that very few boys surveyed appear to have perceived any negative feelings on the part of their first sexual partner. But this is perhaps not surprising, given that only a third of boys have sex more than once with their initial partner. By contrast, a full 57% of the girls who are having sex are going steady with their partner and more than 30% are actually planning to marry their boyfriend.

It is clear, then, that sexual stereotypes often play a major role when adolescents do not make mature, informed decisions about their sexual behavior. Psychologist Frank Cox advises teenagers to evaluate their sexual decisions not according to simplistic, generalized beliefs but according to four different kinds of individual principles: personal, social, religious, and psychological. Adolescents should remember that their emotional and spiritual needs are at least as important as are their physical urges and should play a part in every decision regarding sexual behavior. By acting in ways that harmonize with their personal values, adolescents can enhance their development; by denying or ignoring their values, they risk hindering their own growth.

Another facet of adolescence that requires wisdom and maturity is dealing with alcohol and drugs. Many adolescents develop serious alcohol and drug problems because of the feeling that "everybody's doing it." One 1980 study, "Adolescent Development and the Onset of Drinking," by University of Colorado psychologist Richard Jessor, found that a third of high school and college seniors in the United States could be classified as

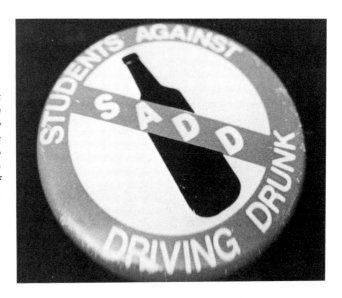

A button for Students Against Drunk Driving (SADD). Studies show that teenagers who drink alcohol excessively are more likely to engage in other forms of rebellious behavior.

problem drinkers, with an even higher rate among first-year male college students. Jessor also found that adolescents who drank heavily were more likely to engage in other rebellious behaviors, such as delinquency, smoking marijuana, and having sexual relations. They also put less value on doing well in school. The converse was also true. Students who engaged in more frequent casual sex were more likely to use alcohol or drugs and to be more influenced by their peers than by their parents' values.

These statistics provide some explanation for why adults often link teenage "problem" behaviors together. Most adolescents become physically mature during their high school years, yet they are granted few adult rights and privileges during this time. As a result, Jessor contends, they search for available ways of "being an adult" or having new experiences. The media bombards adolescents daily with messages of how sexual activity and "partying"—often with beer in hand—allow one to reach the height of sophistication. Unfortunately, many adolescents adopt such messages whole from the magazine page or the movie screen without considering whether these behaviors are personally appropriate for them. Again, the key to making good decisions is to continually examine one's own individual situation and not do whatever other people are doing just because they are doing it.

At the same time, however, it is crucial to recognize that each person is subject to certain basic physical facts regarding "adult" behaviors. A good example here is the use of birth control. A staggering 60% of teenagers engaging in sexual relations do not consistently use any form of contraception. There is no doubt that this statistic is due in large part to a lack of education; some teenagers are unaware that sexual intercourse can indeed result in pregnancy. This high level of nonuse also stems in part from the frequent adolescent belief that "even if other people get pregnant, I won't." Yet pregnancy is something from which no fertile woman is exempt. And indeed, the high rates of teenage pregnancy in America today are a testimony to the fallacy of believing that one can avoid pregnancy without consistent use of birth control.

A study by C. M. Zelnik and J. F. Kantner, published in the journal *Family Planning Perspectives* in 1978, showed that fewer than one-quarter of the unwed teenage mothers surveyed had wanted to have a child, yet only one-fifth had used any form of contraception. And an article in the *Journal of the American Medical Association* by Robert Blum, director of the Adolescent Health Program at the University of Minnesota, claimed that 1

A couple that has planned a pregnancy generally has an easier time raising its child than does a teenage girl who becomes pregnant accidentally.

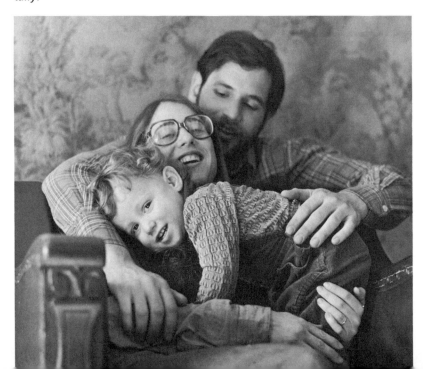

in every 10 adolescent girls in the United States will have an unplanned pregnancy. Studies have shown that these adolescent parents have a lower chance of finishing their education or getting a good job than do their peers who are not parents, and many end up living in poverty.

An American teenager faced with an unplanned pregnancy has three options: She may have the child and keep it herself, have the child and give it up for adoption, or have an abortion. A girl who decides to keep her child will have a much greater chance of coming through unscathed if she is able to reorganize her life after the pregnancy, if she has a good relationship with the father of the child, or if her family is willing to offer support in caring for her baby. Of course, all of these are more likely to occur if the pregnancy is a planned one.

Sexually active teenage girls can receive information about birth control from *gynecologists*, doctors specializing in women's health, who can prescribe birth control pills or fit girls for diaphragms. Many girls are scared about visiting a gynecologist for the first time. In fact, checkups are not only important for maintaining one's health but are usually brief and rarely difficult to go through. Normally, the doctor or nurse practitioner will take a Pap smear, a scraping from the surface of the cervix, to check for cervical cancer. He or she can also offer treatment and advice for less dangerous problems such as the extremely common vaginal yeast infection.

Another situation that can often be avoided with sensible planning, protection, and gynecological advice is the contraction of a *sexually transmitted disease* (STD). As with pregnancy, young people often mistakenly consider themselves immune to these problems, but in fact more than half of all cases of STDs occur during adolescence or the early adult years.

By far the most well publicized and dangerous STD is *acquired immune deficiency syndrome* (AIDS), a fatal disease for which no known cure exists. AIDS is almost always transmitted through sexual contact or the sharing of needles used to inject intravenous drugs. All teenagers who engage in sexual activity need to be aware of "safe sex" methods, such as using a condom, to reduce the risk of AIDS. Although the media initially focused on the outbreak of AIDS among homosexuals, the disease can also be transmitted through intimate contact between members of the opposite sex.

A number of other STDs exist, including syphilis, gonorrhea, chlamydia, and genital warts. These illnesses are all transmitted by sexual contact and can have potentially life-threatening consequences. Most of these potential complications can be avoided, however, if the diseases are recognized and treated in an early stage. Adolescents need to realize that although an STD may seem embarrassing or frightening, it should not be ignored in the hope that it will simply "go away" and the teenager will not have to tell anyone about it. It is particularly important to inform one's sexual partner, but the adolescent should also consult his or her own physician as soon as possible.

Perhaps even more upsetting than the risk of STDs is the violent act of *acquaintance rape*. A shocking number of American adolescent girls have been forced to have sex against their will by someone they know personally. Acquaintance rape is by far the most common form of sexual assault on teenagers; a 1983 study by Suzanne S. Ageton of the Behavioral Research Institute in Boulder, Colorado, found that 50% of teenage rape survivors had been attacked by a date, 30% by a friend, and 11% by a steady boyfriend.

What is particularly disturbing about acquaintance rape is that its high incidence in this country derives not from bizarre criminal impulses but from the same sexual stereotypes that affect much normal teenage dating. Four researchers from the University of California at Los Angeles surveyed 432 teenagers in 1988 and found that more than half of the boys and more than a quarter of the girls considered it proper for a boy to force a girl to have sex if she "led him on" or got him aroused; 43% of the boys and 32% of the girls considered forced sex appropriate simply if the couple had been dating for a long time. Given a number of acquaintance rape scenarios, both sexes also consistently attributed some measure of "fault" for what happened to the girl.

These misguided beliefs have not only contributed to the high number of acquaintance rapes in general but have also made the aftereffects of these crimes particularly devastating for teenage rape survivors. The effects of rape on anyone are often severe, but an adolescent girl in particular may have extreme difficulty

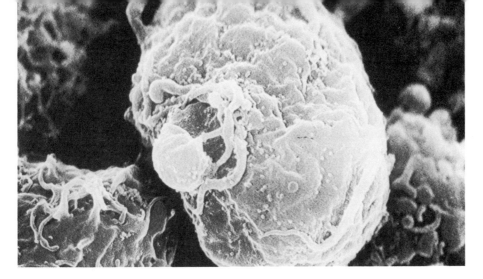

The AIDS virus. AIDS can be transmitted through using contaminated needles to inject intravenous drugs and through sexual intercourse.

coping with such an event coming just when she is struggling to build a strong adult identity for herself. Being a survivor of rape can counteract many important steps in the adolescent growth process and can lead to diminished self-worth, a feeling that no one can be trusted, and negative feelings in general about the outcome of sex and relationships.

Worst of all, if the attacker is a schoolmate of the victimized girl, he may actually brag about the event at school. Because society often applauds the aggressively sexual male and considers rape victims to blame for their experience, the exploits of a teenage rapist may well be celebrated by his peers, whereas the girl will often be ostracized. Indeed, most girls do not tell their parents about an acquaintance rape, usually because of concern that they will be blamed for what happened or for engaging in what their parents may consider inappropriate behavior, such as dating or drinking.

Many victims of acquaintance rape are in fact under the influence of alcohol or drugs when the incident occurs; this might not only impair their judgment about the potential danger of the situation but also may make them less able to resist an unwelcome advance. It should be stressed that being drunk does not make the incident any more a girl's "fault"; no one should ever be coerced into having sex against his or her will. But teenage girls should be aware of the possible dangers of getting themselves too drunk to defend themselves in an acquaintance rape situation.

Much contemporary adolescent behavior is a by-product of the modern era, with its particular values and beliefs. Indeed, the 1960s, 1970s, and 1980s have brought a number of significant changes in Western society that have had major effects on the lives of adolescents. Although certain physical changes will always occur during this period, other changes, such as psychological ones, may differ greatly as society itself adapts to changing times.

•   •   •   •

CHAPTER 6

AMERICAN
ADOLESCENTS
TODAY

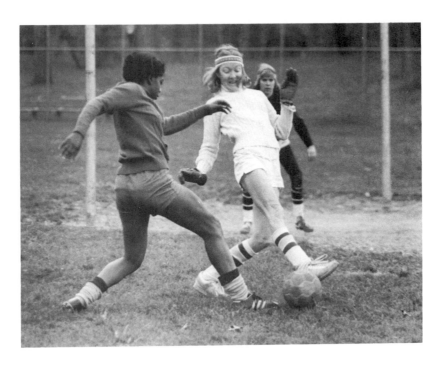

In 1972, the American psychologist Robert Havighurst published a list of eight developmental "tasks" associated with adolescence. Havighurst's premise was that each stage of development can be characterized by certain tasks—that is, events that must occur or goals that must be reached before an individual can successfully enter the next stage. Such tasks, Havighurst claimed, generally fall "midway between an individual need and a societal demand."

Many psychologists agree that Havighurst's developmental tasks are a good way to study the passage through adolescence in modern Western cultures. Part of the tasks' strength as a theory about adolescent growth is that although they may require different kinds of actions or preparation in different stages, their underlying themes are very basic and are in many ways as appropriate today as they were in 1972. Still, it is worth taking a look at how modern conditions of adolescent life in the United States may affect how Havighurst's developmental tasks are thought about and carried out today.

Half of the subjects of the tasks have already been touched upon in previous chapters. These include the following: forming more mature relationships with peers of both sexes (Chapter 4); accepting the body and using it effectively (Chapter 2); preparing for sexual relationships, marriage, and family life (Chapter 5); and acquiring a set of ethics as a guide to behavior (Chapters 3 and 4). This chapter will focus on the four remaining tasks, all of which raise particularly interesting questions today. These are: achieving a masculine or feminine social role; achieving emotional independence from parents and other adults; selecting and preparing for an occupation; and acquiring social literacy.

ACHIEVING A MASCULINE OR FEMININE SOCIAL ROLE

The concept that certain social roles apply only to men and others apply only to women has changed a great deal in the second half of the 20th century. Old-fashioned social roles—men as breadwinners and women as homemakers—have given way to new, more flexible images of the sexes. Today, many women work at salaried jobs outside the home, and many men are responsible for housework or for taking care of children.

Because roles are changing, however, does not mean that Havighurst's task of "achieving a masculine or feminine social role" is an outdated one. Each growing person must still develop a comfortable degree of identification with the social role of one sex or the other. But the definition of what this "social role" entails has changed. More and more, its boundaries are widening,

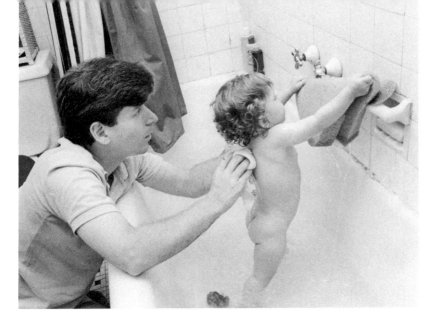

Traditional social roles are becoming obsolete as more women are holding responsible jobs and more men are staying home with their children.

and thus a boy or girl can engage in a greater range of activities while still feeling comfortable about being a boy or a girl.

In earlier times, for example, a teenage girl who enjoyed playing soccer might well have been brought up to believe that sports were masculine, and thus she would probably have given up her interest in soccer in order to conform to society's notion of a feminine social role. Today, a girl is less likely to have received the message that soccer is a gender-related activity, and thus she will be able to feel comfortable in both being a girl and participating in this particular sport.

It is important to understand, however, that "achieving a masculine or feminine social role" does not always mean accepting the roles provided by others. Thus, the girl who has been taught that soccer is a masculine sport may still decide that she can play it and feel "feminine" because her own definition of this term does not exclude playing soccer. Another way for her to come to terms with this interest might be for her to agree that soccer is a male activity but to assert that she, as a girl, nevertheless takes pleasure in this masculine sport; such a girl might think of herself as a tomboy, a girl who acts like a boy. This word is fast becoming outdated, however, as fewer and fewer girls feel obliged to define themselves as "unfeminine" when they engage in traditionally male activities.

In understanding these shifts, it is necessary to realize that the terms *masculine* and *feminine* do not have absolute definitions; they are constantly shaped by what is considered appropriate by society. Sociologists often underscore this fact by making a distinction between "sex," referring to biological difference, and "gender," which is often defined as the societal differences that are imposed on men and women without necessarily being based on biological facts.

Like all of Havighurst's tasks, this particular one requires a balance between "individual needs" and "societal demands." The expectations of society need not dictate how teenagers perceive themselves, but they should be aware of what those expectations may be. Thus, a boy who takes up a traditionally feminine activity, such as dance, should recognize that some people may have difficulty accepting his decision and may question his "masculinity" along the way. As long as he has accepted that he can

Teenagers often mistakenly classify some activities as exclusively feminine and others as strictly masculine. In truth, however, boys who dance—and girls who play sports—can do so and maintain their own sexual identity.

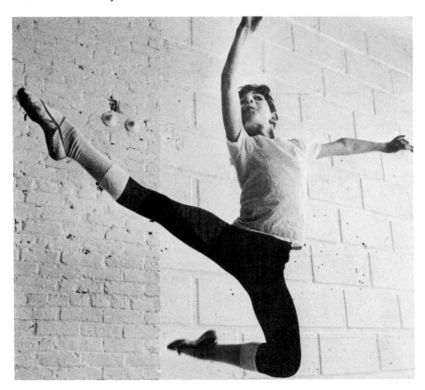

be a boy and still enjoy dancing, however, he has fulfilled Havighurst's requirement and need only rely on his own acceptance of himself as a means of standing up to the differing viewpoints of others.

ACHIEVING EMOTIONAL INDEPENDENCE FROM PARENTS AND ADULTS

As discussed in Chapter 4, an important part of adolescent growth involves learning to rely less on parents or other adults for all of one's needs. Adolescents who successfully complete this task will begin to make more of their own decisions and to take pride in their achievements for their own sake rather than because they are rewarded by their parents' approval. This process is sometimes called *desatellization* because it draws the adolescent out of the "satellite" position in emotional orbit around the parents. It usually begins around age 12 or age 13 and does not end until about age 21.

This particular developmental task, however, has also changed somewhat in the 1970s and 1980s. In 1960, 1 out of every 10 American children lived with only 1 parent; in 1985, the ratio had skyrocketed to 1 in 5. This change has been the result of rising rates of both divorce and unwed parenthood. In addition, many children who live with only their mother may see her much less frequently than in the past, because she is more likely to have a full-time job outside the home. Because of the difficulty of supporting a child on one income, many single mothers may have to work especially hard simply to feed, clothe, and shelter their family.

Many people have criticized these changes in the traditional American family, believing that having mothers who work or parents who divorce can only be harmful to children. Research has not borne this out, however. An extensive series of studies by the Washington, D.C.–based Panel on Work, Family, and Community in 1983 found no consistent effects on a child's development or educational success if his or her mother worked. And teenagers themselves provide further evidence that a working mother does not lead to an unhappy adolescence: 70% of the boys and girls interviewed by Jane Norman and Myron W. Harris claimed to be happy that their mother worked, citing such reasons as the mother's own happiness and her feeling of freedom, as well the necessity of her earning an income.

Despite the trauma involved, most adolescents maintained even in the case of divorce that the end result was a positive one. Seventy-five percent of the teenagers interviewed by Norman and Harris felt that a divorce was preferable to an unhappy marital situation. Nearly one-third felt that living with 1 parent meant less of a "hassle," and an additional 18% claimed that they did not think about it much at all. Only 9% felt embarrassed or "different" for living with only 1 parent. Although nearly half of the adolescents in the study did say that they missed their other parent or hoped their parents would get back together, the results show that such feelings did not usually imply that the teenagers felt the divorce had been a mistake.

Although psychologists are still vigorously debating the long-term effects of living with one parent, most agree that young people whose parents divorce generally must deal with more responsibility and more time alone than do adolescents whose parents remain happily married. For teenagers of divorce, then, Havighurst's task of "achieving independence from the family" may become a necessity earlier than for others.

Whether this speeding up of a basic process leads to an increased sense of maturity and capability or to confusion and worry will depend largely on the support that the adolescent in a single-parent home receives from siblings, friends, and other adults as well as from the parent who remains. Trust, patience, and open communication between parent and child can turn the experience into a valuable one that can have a positive effect on growth. But avoiding the new issues raised by divorce may well lead to feelings of doubt, misunderstanding, and uncertainty, and instead of growing up faster the adolescent may feel less able to deal with new responsibility.

SELECTING AND PREPARING FOR AN OCCUPATION

When Havighurst uses the word occupation, he refers to the employment that an individual will have as an adult. It is important to recognize also, however, that in contemporary American society a great number of adolescents also work during their high school years. Psychologists Ellen Greenberger and Lawrence Steinberg, who researched this phenomenon in their book *When Teenagers Work*, see this as a "distinctly American phenomenon." In Europe, where fewer opportunities for higher education exist and competition for a place in college can be fierce, adolescents often spend more time on their schoolwork than American teenagers do and thus may have trouble holding down a job while still in school.

In the United States, Greenberger and Steinberg argue, working during one's school years is considered not only normal but, by many adults, a positive experience for young people. These adults stress the experience of having responsibility, of making money to help support the family, and, because one of an adult's chief tasks is working at a job, of acting more like an adult. Because of these factors, many adults consider teenagers who work to be more mature.

Greenberger and Steinberg argue against this view of adolescent labor, however. Their findings indicate that teenage employment, although beneficial for some, often interferes with schoolwork, promotes luxury spending, correlates with delinquent behavior such as substance abuse, and leads not to respect for the idea of a job but to increased cynicism about it. They warn that adolescents are capable of playing adult roles in a superficial way without truly having achieved maturity and self-understanding. Indeed, Erik Erikson, who wrote of the need during adolescence for a *psychosocial moratorium*, a period of relative freedom from responsibility, worried that working during these crucial years could take time away from the important tasks of growth that help an adolescent to mature.

Of course, some adolescents work because their family truly needs the extra income to survive. But Greenberger and Steinberg found that this was rarely the case; fewer than 10% of the teenagers they studied contributed "a substantial amount" of their income to their family. Part of the reason for this low percentage, however, may be that poor or underprivileged adolescents often have difficulty finding jobs at all. Indeed, Greenberger and Steinberg stressed that a much greater number of black and Hispanic young people seek—rather than have—a job than do white adolescents.

This distinction points out an important difference in the experience of American adolescents who begin to think about a job for themselves both as young people and in their life as an adult. In recent years, the increasing use of computers and other forms of high technology in many jobs has meant that few young people today are able to enter the job market without extending their skills beyond the high school level. But college is often a considerable expense, one that many families cannot afford.

For those adolescents who do attend college, the cost forces many to remain financially dependent upon their parents for a good deal longer than they would have otherwise. These young people may continue to live at home to save money after they begin job training or work; thus, they may postpone marrying and starting a family for a few years while they complete their schooling or look for work. This delay in beginning an independent financial and social life may be linked to a delay in reaching emotional independence. In 1988, psychologist Susan J. Frank of Michigan State University reported in the journal *Developmental Psychology* that until as late as ages 24 to 28, most young adults continue to rely on their parents to make important choices in their life and feel unable to cope with problems without help from their parents. Today, said Frank in a *New York Times* interview, "adolescence doesn't really end until the late 20s."

But the idea that adolescents mature more slowly because of the increasing amount of time needed to prepare for a job is not accurate in all cases. Many teenagers of lower socioeconomic status are unable to afford expensive job training or are staying at home and straining their parents' already modest income. A devastating statistic of the late 1980s has been the rising rate of children who live in poverty; one out of every five U.S. children is now poor, and in 1984 half of these poor children lived in households headed by a single mother. Factors such as the lack of adequate child support and inequitable wages for women, especially minority women, have contributed to a general problem of poverty in female-headed households. It seems unlikely that the teenage children of these women will be able to postpone their adolescent task of finding a job and leaving home because of the already significant burden on their mother.

Given the increasing use of sophisticated technology, such as computers, in the workplace, many poor adolescents will be shut out of the training required even for entry-level jobs. For poor black teenagers, the additional burden of racism may make the search even harder. A study by A. Ziajka in 1972 found that black adolescents often see themselves as less valuable, less important, less able, and less responsible than do whites of a similar age. The blacks studied also frequently saw the outside world as hostile toward them.

All of these feelings can create severe handicaps for black adolescents who need to fulfill Havighurst's tasks to succeed in American society. The issue of finding a job is only one particularly troublesome problem for young people whose living situation and life experience has led them to believe that they have nothing to offer or that society has no interest in them. Such youths may experience a certain form of "prolonged adolescence" because fulfilling Havighurst's tasks will be difficult for them, but this is hardly a luxury or the result of privilege.

ACQUIRING SOCIAL LITERACY

Acquiring social literacy, the last of Havighurst's tasks, is also one that needs to be examined in light of racial and socioeconomic differences. Again, Havighurst's general definition of the task was a broad one: "Socially literate" means being able to get along in society in a basic way. This entails understanding and being able to apply such skills as working effectively with others in a group. Havighurst claimed that this task begins in later adolescence, around age 17 or 18, and that it is never truly completed; it continues throughout life.

It can be said that there are basic social skills that every member of society should have. But it is difficult to define exactly what "social literacy" means because different situations can call for vastly different responses. Adolescents—for example, poor or minority teenagers—who grow up on the fringes of what is generally thought of as "mainstream American society" may have learned ways of dealing with others that prove as successful for them as do entirely different approaches for white or middle-class youths. These modes of behavior may be based on a different field of knowledge entirely, as demonstrated by the sociologist A. Dove, who created a test designed to point out how standard tests of intelligence are biased toward white students. Dove called his exam "the chitling test"; its questions were designed to reflect the language and experiences of the black ghetto, and many white adolescents would be hard put to answer them. Thus, Dove called attention to the differences in what is considered culturally significant for blacks and for whites. If such differences exist, who can define a general form of social literacy?

Gradually, Americans are beginning to accept the importance of recognizing cultural diversity. College courses have begun to place new emphasis on women, blacks, and non-American cultures in an effort to expand students' horizons instead of limiting them to one general view of what is important to know. Certain basic requirements remain for all levels of schooling, but in general the 1980s have seen a broadening in how social literacy is defined. In order to fulfill the task of acquiring social literacy in the modern age, adolescents will need to be increasingly aware of perspectives and life experiences beyond what they have experienced themselves.

ADOLESCENTS AROUND THE WORLD

In 1986, the *United Nations Chronicle* announced that the number of people between the ages of 15 and 19 was expected to reach 1 billion by 1990 and 1.3 billion by 2025. Its report also listed some likely trends among adolescents: increasing unemployment and underemployment of youth; a growing gap between the education provided by school systems and the needs of the workplace; and a weakening of the bonds between young people and their family as outside forces such as peers and the media gain increasing influence.

According to "Situation of Youth in the 1980s," a report issued by the UN, the adolescents of the world numbered 922 million in 1985. This means that young people account for one-fifth of the global population. Sadly, a staggering number of these adolescents—fully 80% of them, up from 69% in 1950—live in developing nations that are troubled by poverty, disease, hunger, unemployment, and lack of social services. And this trend is likely to continue. Since 1970, the percentage of the world youth population living in Latin America, South Asia, and Africa, where many poor nations are concentrated, has steadily increased. African nations in particular will probably experience a surge in the growth of their adolescent population during the 1990s. By contrast, the percentage of youths living in North America, Europe, and the Soviet Union has decreased since 1970, while the number in East Asia and the Pacific region has remained fairly steady.

These demographic projections have serious implications for the lives of millions of young people. Studies reported in 1988 in *The Teenage World: Adolescents' Self-image in Ten Countries*, by Daniel Offer, Eric Ostrov, and Kenneth I. Howard, suggested that a direct relationship exists between a nation's gross national product (GNP)—a measure of its overall prosperity—and the emotional well-being of its adolescents. In other words, claimed these authors, the poorer the nation, the more likely it is that a greater proportion of its young people will be seriously affected by sadness, loneliness, and other debilitating emotions. Thus, if the developing nations' share of the world adolescent population continues to rise, the incidence of adolescent emotional distress around the world is likely to rise as well.

The authors of *The Teenage World* also point out that certain social and mental health problems have been linked to birth cohort size—that is, to the proportion of adolescents in a population. (A birth cohort includes everyone born within a particular set of years, such as the much discussed "baby boom" generation born during the 1950s in the United States.) For example, the suicide rate among adolescents has been shown to increase in populations where adolescents have a larger birth cohort. This finding too points to difficulty for less developed countries, where families tend to be larger for a number of reasons—not least among them the fact that children often die at an early age from malnutrition or untreated disease, and thus to ensure having five healthy children often means bearing as many as ten.

Another concern facing tomorrow's adolescents is employment. A lack of jobs is already one of the most serious problems young people face around the world, and unemployment is only expected to increase, according to the UN report. Today's birth rate determines the number of people who will be entering the job market in 15 or 20 years; in nearly all the developing nations, people are being born at a much higher rate than jobs are being created. Especially in Africa, where drought and agricultural problems have depressed the economy over much of the continent, unemployment among the young is likely to skyrocket well into the 21st century. Even in Western Europe, where the ratio of adolescents in the population has remained fairly stable since 1970 and where the percentage of adolescents who receive a complete education is higher than in any other region, unemployment among adolescents who wish to work and young adults entering the labor force is as high as 40% to 50% in some countries because of economic stagnation and competition for the few available jobs.

On the brighter side, young people everywhere are being increasingly affected by the rapid pace of cultural change and by the way in which immigration, travel, and the media are bringing many different cultures into contact with one another. These changes are evident in the extent to which Havighurst's developmental tasks have taken on new meanings in contemporary American society as traditional considerations about gender roles, the family, and social literacy begin to shift and often to widen.

The authors of *The Teenage World* found that teenagers from widely differing cultural backgrounds had, as they said, "more in common than might have been thought to be the case." They suggested that a sense of unity and commonality among the world's adolescents, now on the verge of adulthood, could lead to new forms of cooperation and creative problem solving that may ease the way for the adolescents of tomorrow.

•   •   •   •

APPENDIX:
FOR MORE INFORMATION

The following is a list of organizations that can provide further information on issues related to adolescence.

GENERAL

American Mental Health
  Foundation
2 East 86th Street
New York, NY 10028
(212) 737-9027

Canadian Mental Health
  Association
2160 Yonge Street
Toronto, Ontario M4F 2Z3
Canada
(416) 484-7750

Carnegie Council on Adolescent
  Development
c/o Carnegie Corporation of New
  York
437 Madison Avenue
New York, NY 10022
(212) 371-3200

Center for Early Adolescence
Carr Mill Mall
Suite 211
University of North Carolina at
  Chapel Hill
Carrboro, NC 27510
(919) 966-1148

National Collaboration for Youth
1319 F Street NW
Suite 601
Washington, DC 20004
(202) 347-2080

National Health Information Center
Office of Disease Prevention and
  Health Promotion
U.S. Department of Health and
  Human Services
P.O. Box 1133
Washington, DC 20013-1133
(800) 336-4797
(301) 565-4167

Society for Adolescent Medicine
Suite 120
19401 East 40 Highway
Independence, MO 64455
(816) 795-TEEN
(provides a list of health care
  professionals associated with the
  organization and a list of
  adolescent clinics throughout the
  United States and Canada)

ALCOHOL AND DRUG ABUSE

Al-Anon
Family Group Headquarters
Box 862
Midtown Station
New York, NY 10018
(212) 302-7240
(for nearest chapter consult your
  local telephone white pages)

85

Alcohol/Drug Abuse Referral
Hotline:(800) ALCOHOL

Alcoholics Anonymous
Box 459
Grand Central Annex
New York, NY 10017

Care Unit National Treatment
System
410 South Tustin Avenue
Orange, CA 92666
(800) 556-CARE

Cocaine Anonymous
World Service Office
Box 1367
Culver City, CA 90239
Hot Line in Los Angeles:
(213) 839-1141

National Association of Children of
Alcoholics
31706 Coast Highway
Suite 201
South Laguna, CA 92677
(714) 499-3889

National Hotline for Cocaine
Information and Help:
(800) COCAINE

National Institute on Alcohol Abuse
and Alcoholism
5600 Fisher Lane
Rockville, MD 20857

National Institute on Drug Abuse
5600 Fishers Lane
Rockville, MD 20857
(800) 662-HELP

DEPRESSION

Depression Anonymous Recovery
from Depression
329 East 62nd Street
New York, NY 10021
(212) 689-2600

Manic Depressive Association of
Metropolitan Toronto
40 Orchard View Boulevard
Suite 252
Toronto, Ontario M4R 1B9
Canada
(416) 486-8046

National Depressive and Manic-
Depressive Association
222 South Riverside Plaza
Suite 2812
Chicago, IL 60606
(312) 993-0066

EATING DISORDERS

American Anorexia and Bulimia
Association
133 Cedar Lane
Teaneck, NJ 07666
(201) 836-1800

Glenbeigh Food Addictions Hot
Line
(800) 4A-BINGE

National Anorexic Aid Society
5796 Karl Road
Columbus, OH 43229
(614) 436-1112

National Association of Anorexia
Nervosa and Associated
Disorders
Box 7
Highland Park, IL 60035
(312) 831-3438

Overeaters Anonymous
World Service Office
4025 Spencer Street, #203
Torrance, California 90503
Mail address: P.O. Box 92870
Los Angeles, CA 90009
(213) 542-8363

HOMOSEXUALITY

Institute for the Protection of
Lesbian and Gay Youth, Inc.
110 East 23rd Street
10th Floor
New York, NY 10010
(212) 473-1113

Gay Switchboard Hot Line
(national referrals)
(215) 546-7100

National Federation of Parents and
Friends of Gays
8020 Eastern Avenue NW
Washington, DC 20012
(202) 726-3223

PREGNANCY AND PARENTHOOD

National Association Concerned
with School-Age Parents
7315 Wisconsin Avenue
Suite 211-W
Washington, DC 20014
(write for group nearest you)

National Women's Health Network
224 7th Street SE
Washington, DC 20003
(202) 543-9222

Planned Parenthood Federation of
America
810 7th Avenue
New York, NY 10019
(212) 541-7800

RAPE

National Clearinghouse on Marital
and Date Rape
2325 Oak Street
Berkeley, CA 94708
(415) 548-1770

Sexual Abuse Hotline:
(202) 333-RAPE

(emergency counseling for rape
victims offering medical
information and referrals to local
treatment and support groups)

SEXUALLY TRANSMITTED DISEASES

American College Health
Association
15879 Crabbs Branch Way
Rockville, MD 20855

American Social Health Association
260 Sheridan Avenue
Palo Alto, CA 94306

Herpes Resource Center
P.O. Box 100
Palo Alto, CA 94306
(415) 321-5134

National AIDS Center
Health Protection Building, B7
Tunney's Pasture
Ottawa, Ontario K1A 1B4
Canada
(613) 957-1774

National Sexually Transmitted
Diseases Hotline
(800) 227-8922

U.S. Public Health Service
Office of Public Affairs
Hubert H. Humphrey Building
Room 725-H
200 Independence Avenue SW
Washington, DC 20201
National AIDS Hot Line:
(800) 342-AIDS

SUICIDE

American Association of
Suicidology
2459 South Ash Street
Denver, CO 80222
(provides state listing of suicide
prevention centers and hot lines)
(303) 692-0985

ADOLESCENCE

Canadian Association on Suicide
Prevention
c/o Dr. Antoon A. Leenaars
3366 Dandurand Boulevard
Windsor, Ontario N9E 2E8
Canada
(519) 253-9377

Suicide Information and Education
Center
Suite 201
1615 Tenth Avenue SW
Calgary, Alberta T3C 0J7
Canada, (403) 245-3900
Crisis Phone: (403) 266-1605

The following is a list of adolescent clinics in the United States and Canada.

UNITED STATES

ALABAMA

Children's Hospital
Adolescent Clinic
1600 Seventh Avenue, South
Birmingham, AL 35233
(205) 939-9100

ARIZONA

Arizona Health Sciences Center
Adolescent Clinic
1501 North Campbell Avenue

Tucson, AZ 85724
(602) 626-6629

St. Joseph's Hospital
Adolescent Unit
P.O. Box 2071
Phoenix, AZ 85006
(602) 241-3160

ARKANSAS

Adolescent Youth Clinic
Children's Hospital
800 Marshall Street
Little Rock, AR 72202
(501) 370-1420

CALIFORNIA

Adolescent Clinic
Children's Hospital
3700 California Street
San Francisco, CA 94119
(415) 387-8700

Teenage Health Clinic
Children's Hospital
4650 Sunset Boulevard
Los Angeles, CA 90027
(213) 669-2153

COLORADO

University of Colorado Medical
Center
Adolescent Clinic
4200 East Ninth Avenue
Denver, CO 80220
(303) 394-8461

Westside Teen Clinic
990 Federal Boulevard
Second Floor
Denver, CO 80204
(303) 592-7401

CONNECTICUT

Adolescent Clinic
Hartford Hospital
80 Ceymour Street
Hartford, CT 06115
(203) 524-3011

Adolescent Unit
Bridgeport Hospital
267 Grant Street
Bridgeport, CT 06602
(203) 384-3064

DELAWARE

Alfred I. duPont Institute
P.O. Box 269
Wilmington, DE 19899
(302) 651-4000

DISTRICT OF COLUMBIA

Child & Youth Services
Georgetown University
3800 Reservoir Road
Washington, DC 20007
(202) 625-7452

Department of Adolescent Medicine
Children's Hospital, National
111 Michigan Avenue NW
Washington, DC 20010
(202) 576-1107

FLORIDA

Adolescent Health Care Service
University of Miami School of
  Medicine
P.O. Box 01620 (D-820)
Miami, FL 33101
(305) 547-5880

HAWAII

Adolescent Program
Kapiolani Children's Medical
  Center
1319 Punahou Street
Honolulu, HI 96826
(808) 947-8511

Adolescent Unit
Straub Clinic and Hospital
888 South King Street
Honolulu, HI 96813
(808) 523-2311

ILLINOIS

Adolescent Clinic
Michael Reese Hospital
29th Street at Ellis Avenue
Chicago, IL 60616
(312) 791-2000

Adolescent Clinic
Rush-Presbyterian Hospital
1753 West Congress Parkway
Chicago, IL 60612
(312) 942-5000

IOWA

Adolescent Clinic
Departments of Medicine and
  Pediatrics
University of Iowa Hospitals
Iowa City, IA 52242
(319) 356-2229

KENTUCKY

Adolescent Clinic/Adolescent GYN
  Clinic
Division of Adolescent Medicine
Norton Children's Hospital
Louisville, KY 40202
(502) 562-8836
(502) 562-7765

LOUISIANA

Adolescent Medical and Surgical
  Unit
Touro Infirmary
1401 Foucher Street
New Orleans, LA 70115
(504) 897-7011

Adolescent Program
East Jefferson General Hospital
4200 Houma Boulevard
Metairie, LA 70011
(504) 454-4000

MARYLAND

Adolescent Clinic
Montgomery County Health
  Department
8500 Colesville Road
Silver Spring, MD 20910
(301) 565-7729

Adolescent Program
Johns Hopkins University
Broadway at Orleans Street
Baltimore, MD 21205
(301) 955-5000

MICHIGAN

Adolescent Ambulatory Service
Children's Hospital
3901 Beaubien Boulevard
Detroit, MI 48201
(313) 494-5762

Internal/Adolescent Medicine
Out-Patient Building
University Hospital
Ann Arbor, MI 48109
(313) 763-5170

MINNESOTA

Adolescent Health Diagnostic Clinic
University Hospital
Harvard Street at East River Road
Minneapolis, MN 55455
(612) 626-2820

Teenage Medical Services
2425 Chicago Avenue
Minneapolis, MN 55404
(612) 874-6125

MISSISSIPPI

Adolescent Medicine Services
Keesler Air Force Base Medical
  Center
Keesler AFB, MS 39534
(601) 377-3766

Rush Clinic
1314 19th Avenue
Meridian, MS 39301
(601) 483-0011

MISSOURI

Adolescent Clinic
Cardinal Glennon Memorial
  Hospital For Children
1465 South Grand
St. Louis, MO 63104
(314) 577-5600

Adolescent Clinic
Children's Mercy Hospital
240 Gillham Road
Kansas City, MO 64108
(816) 234-3000

MONTANA

Department of Adolescence
Great Falls Clinic
1220 Central Avenue
Great Falls, MT 59409
(406) 454-2171

NEBRASKA

Adolescent Clinic
Omaha Children's Hospital
12808 Augusta Avenue
Omaha, NE 68144
(402) 330-5690

NEW JERSEY

Adolescent Clinic
Monmouth Medical Center
Long Branch, NJ 07740
(201) 222-5200

Adolescent Services and Clinic
Morristown Memorial Hospital
100 Madison Avenue
Morristown, NJ 07960
(201) 540-5199

NEW YORK

Adolescent Clinic
601 Elmwood Avenue
Rochester, NY 14642
(716) 275-2962

Adolescent Clinic
New York Hospital
525 East 68th Street
New York, NY 10021
(212) 472-5454

NORTH CAROLINA

Duke University Medical Center
Youth Clinic, Department of
  Pediatrics
Durham, NC 27710
(919) 684-3872

Wake County Medical Center
Adolescent Clinic
3000 New Bern Road
Raleigh, NC 27610
(919) 755-8521

NORTH DAKOTA

Fargo Clinic
737 Broadway
Fargo, ND 58102
(701) 237-2431

OHIO

Adolescent Clinic
Cleveland Metro. General Hospital
3395 Scranton Road
Cleveland, OH 44109
(216) 398-6000

Adolescent Clinic
Pavilion Building
Children's Hospital Medical Center
Elland and Bethesda Avenues
Cincinnati, OH 45229
(513) 559-4681

OKLAHOMA

Adolescent Medicine Clinic
Children's Memorial Hospital
940 North East 13th Street
Oklahoma City, OK 73190
(405) 271-4371

Adolescent Medicine Program
University of Oklahoma
2815 South Sheridan Road
Tulsa, OK 74129
(918) 838-4823

PENNSYLVANIA

Adolescent Medical Center
1723 Woodbourne Road
Suite 10
Levittown, PA 19057
(215) 946-8353

SOUTH CAROLINA

Adolescent Clinic
Greenville General Hospital
701 Grove Road
Greenville, SC 29605
(803) 242-8625

Medical Park Pediatrics and
  Adolescent Clinic

3321 Park Road
Columbia, SC 29203
(803) 779-7380

TEXAS

Adolescent Clinic
Children's Medical Center
1935 Amelia Street
Dallas, TX 75235
(214) 637-3820

Adolescent Clinic of Texas
Children's Hospital
6621 Fannin Street, Room 0109
Houston, TX 77030
(713) 791-2831

VIRGINIA

Adolescent Health Service
Children's Medical Center
Medical College of Virginia
Box 151 - MCV Station
Richmond, VA 23298
(804) 786-9449

Adolescent Medicine
Children's Hospital of the Kings'
  Daughters
800 West Olney Road
Norfolk, VA 23507
(804) 622-1381

WASHINGTON

Adolescent Clinic
University of Washington
Division of Adolescent Medicine
Seattle, WA 98105
(206) 545-1274

Adolescent Health Clinic
Tacoma Pierce County
Health Department
Tacoma, WA 98405
(206) 593-4100

WISCONSIN

Adolescent Health Center
Milwaukee Children's Hospital
1700 West Wisconsin Avenue
Milwaukee, WI 53233
(414) 931-4105

ADOLESCENCE

Teenage Clinic
Clinical Sciences Center
600 Highland Avenue
Madison, WI 53792
(608) 263-6406

CANADA

ONTARIO

Adolescent Clinic
Hospital for Sick Children
555 University Avenue
Toronto, Ontario M5G 1X8
(416) 597-1500

I.O.D.E. Children's Centre
North York General
4001 Leslie Street
Willowdale, Ontario M2K 1E1
(416) 492-3836

QUEBEC

Adolescent Clinic
Ste-Justin Hospital
3175 Côte Ste-Cathérine
Montreal, Quebec H3T 1C5
(514) 345-4931

Adolescent Unit
Montreal Children's Hospital
2300 Tupper Street
Montreal, Quebec H3H 1P3
(514) 937-8511

Child and Adolescent Services
3666 McTavish Street
Montreal, Quebec H3A 1Y8
(514) 392-5022

Miriam Kennedy Child and Family
  Clinic
509 Pine Avenue, West
Montreal, Quebec H2W 1S4
(514) 849-1315

FURTHER READING

GENERAL

Atwater, Eastwood. *Adolescence.* Englewood Cliffs, NJ: Prentice-Hall, 1983.

Benedict, Ruth. "Continuities and Discontinuities in Cultural Conditioning." *Psychiatry* 1 (1938): 161–67.

Blos, Peter. *The Adolescent Passage.* New York: International Universities Press, 1979.

———. *On Adolescence.* New York: Free Press, 1962.

Cohen, Yehudi. *The Transition from Childhood to Adolescence.* Chicago: Aldine Publishing Co., 1962.

Dacey, John S. *Adolescents Today.* Santa Monica, CA: Goodyear, 1979.

Dobson, James. *Preparing for Adolescence.* New York: Bantam Books, 1980.

Eagan, Andrea Boroff. *Why Am I So Miserable if These Are the Best Years of My Life?: A Survival Guide for the Young Woman.* Philadelphia: Lippincott, 1976.

Fuhrmann, Barbara Schneider. *Adolescence, Adolescents.* Boston: Little, Brown, 1986.

Hall, Granville Stanley. *Adolescence.* 2 vols. New York: Appleton-Century-Crofts, 1904.

Johnson, Eric W. *How to Live Through Junior High School: A Practical Discussion of the Middle and Junior High School Years for Parents, Students, and Teachers.* Philadelphia: Lippincott, 1975.

Kaplan, Louise J. *Adolescence: The Farewell to Childhood.* New York: Simon & Schuster, 1984.

Kiell, Norman. *The Universal Experience of Adolescence.* Boston: Beacon Press, 1967.

Lambert, B. Geraldine. *Adolescence: A Transition from Childhood to Maturity.* Monterey, CA: Brooks/Cole, 1978.

Mitchell, John J. *Human Life: The Early Adolescent Years.* Toronto: Holt, Rinehart & Winston of Canada, 1974.

Muuss, Rolf E. H. *Theories of Adolescence.* New York: Random House, 1968.

Offer, Daniel, Eric Ostrov, and Kenneth Howard. *The Adolescent: A Psychological Self-Portrait.* New York: Basic Books, 1981.

———. *The Teenage World: Adolescents' Self-Image in Ten Countries.* New York: Plenum, 1988.

Simon, Nissa. *Don't Worry, You're Normal: A Teenager's Guide to Self-Health.* New York: Crowell, 1982.

Stevens-Long, Judith, and Nancy J. Cobb. *Adolescence and Early Adulthood.* Palo Alto, CA: Mayfield, 1983.

White, Kathleen M., and Joseph Speisman. *Adolescence.* Monterey, CA: Brooks/Cole, 1977.

PUBERTY AND PHYSICAL DEVELOPMENT

Gilbert, Sara D. *Feeling Good: A Book About You and Your Body.* New York: Four Winds Press, 1978.

Grinder, Robert E. *Studies in Adolescence: A Book of Readings in Adolescent Development.* New York: Macmillan, 1975.

Howells, John G. *Modern Perspectives in Adolescent Psychiatry.* New York: Brunner/Mazel, 1971.

Katchadourian, Herant A. *The Biology of Adolescence.* San Francisco: Freeman, 1977.

Lerner, Richard M., James B. Orlos, and John R. Knapp. "Physical Attractiveness, Physical Effectiveness, and Self-Concept in Late Adolescents." *Adolescence* 11, no. 43 (1976): 313–26.

Lipke, Jeanne Coryllel. *Puberty and Adolescence.* Minneapolis: Lerner, 1971.

Madaras, Lynda. *The What's Happening to My Body Book for Boys: A Growing Up Guide for Parents and Sons.* New York: Newmarket Press, 1984.

Madaras, Lynda, and Area Madaras. *Lynda Madaras' Growing-Up Guide for Girls.* New York: Newmarket Press, 1986.

Sommer, Barbara Baker. *Puberty and Adolescence.* New York: Oxford University Press, 1978.

Tanner, James M. *Foetus into Man: Physical Growth from Conception to Maturity.* Cambridge: Harvard University Press, 1978.

———. *Growth at Adolescence.* 2nd ed. Oxford: Blackwell, 1962.

CHANGES IN EMOTIONS AND THOUGHTS

Adelson, Joseph. *Handbook of Adolescent Psychology.* New York: Wiley, 1980.

Frieze, Irene H., et al. *Women and Sex Roles.* New York: Norton, 1978.

Gallatin, Judith. *Adolescents and Individuality.* New York: Harper & Row, 1975.

Gardner, Sandra. *Teenage Suicide.* New York: Messner, 1985.

LeShan, Eda J. *You and Your Feelings.* New York: Macmillan, 1975.

Lickona, Thomas. *Moral Development and Behavior: Theory, Research, and Social Issues.* New York: Holt, Rinehart & Winston, 1976.

McCandless, Boyd R., and Richard H. Coop. *Adolescents: Behavior and Development.* 2nd ed. New York: Holt, Rinehart & Winston, 1979.

Reingold, Carmel Berman. *How to Cope: A Guide to the Teen-Age Years.* New York: Watts, 1974.

Thornburg, Hershel D. *Development in Adolescence.* Monterey, CA: Brooks/Cole, 1982.

RELATIONSHIPS AND IDENTITY

Balswick, Jack O., and Clitos Macrides. "Parental Stimulus for Adolescent Rebellion." *Adolescence* 10, no. 38 (1975): 253–66.

Conger, John Janeway. *Adolescence: Generation Under Pressure.* New York: Harper & Row, 1979.

———. *Basic and Contemporary Issues in Developmental Psychology.* New York: Harper & Row, 1975.

Cox, Frank. *Human Intimacy: Marriage, the Family, and Its Meaning.* New York: West, 1978.

Curtis, Russell L. "Adolescent Orientations Toward Parents and Peers: Variations by Sex, Age, and Socioeconomic Status." *Adolescence* 10, no. 40 (1975): 483–94.

Gilligan, Carol. *In a Different Voice: Psychological Theory and Women's Development.* Cambridge: Harvard University Press, 1982.

Kandel, D. B. "Similarity in Real-Life Adolescent Friendship Pairs." *Journal of Personality and Social Psychology* 36 (1978): 306–12.

Marks, Jane. *Help! My Parents Are Driving Me Crazy.* New York: Ace Books, 1982.

Rubin, Lillian. *Just Friends: The Role of Friendship in Our Lives.* New York: Harper & Row, 1985.

Skolnick, Arlene. *The Intimate Environment: Exploring Marriage and Family.* 2nd ed. Boston: Little, Brown, 1978.

Thornburg, Hershel D. *Contemporary Adolescence: Readings.* 2nd ed. Monterey, CA: Brooks/Cole, 1975.

TRYING OUT ADULT BEHAVIORS

Bell, Ruth. *Changing Bodies, Changing Lives: A Book for Teens on Sex and Relationships.* New York: Random House, 1980.

Furstenberg, Frank F., Jr. *Teenage Sexuality, Pregnancy and Childbearing.* Philadelphia: University of Pennsylvania Press, 1981.

Hass, Aaron. *Teenage Sexuality: A Survey of Teenage Sexual Behavior.* New York: Macmillan, 1979.

Hettlinger, Richard Frederick. *Growing Up with Sex: A Guide for the Early Teens.* New York: Continuum, 1980.

Muuss, Rolf E. H., *Adolescent Behavior and Society.* 3rd ed. New York: Random House, 1980.

Norman, Jane, and Myron W. Harris, Ph.D. *The Private Life of the American Teenager.* New York: Rowson, Wade, 1981.

Wachter, Oralee. *Sex, Drugs, and AIDS.* New York: Bantam Books, 1987.

Warshaw, Robin. *I Never Called It Rape: The Ms. Report on Recognizing, Fighting, and Surviving Date and Acquaintance Rape.* New York: Harper & Row, 1988.

Zelnik, Melvin, and John F. Kantner. "First Pregnancies to Women Aged 15–19: 1976 and 1971." *Family Planning Perspectives* 10, no. 3 (May/June 1978): 135–42.

AMERICAN ADOLESCENTS TODAY

Children's Defense Fund. *Black and White Children in America: Key Facts.* Washington, DC: Children's Defense Fund, 1985.

Dove, A. "Taking the Chitling Test." *Newsweek,* July 15, 1968.

Elkind, David. *All Grown Up and No Place to Go.* Reading, MA: Addison-Wesley, 1984.

Greenberger, Ellen, and Lawrence Steinberg. *When Teenagers Work: The Psychological and Social Costs of Adolescent Development.* New York: Basic Books, 1986.

Hayes, Cheryl D., and Sheila B. Kamerman, eds. *Children of Working Parents: Experiences and Outcomes.* Washington, DC: National Academy Press, 1983.

Looft, William. *Developmental Psychology: A Book of Readings.* Hillsdale, IL: Dryden, 1972.

Musgrove, Frank. *Youth and the Social Order.* Bloomington: Indiana University Press, 1965.

Rodgers, Harrell R., Jr. *Poor Women, Poor Families: The Economic Plight of America's Female-Headed Households.* Armonk, NY: Sharpe, 1986.

Snedeker, Bonnie. *Hard Knocks: Preparing Youth for Work.* Baltimore: Johns Hopkins University Press, 1982.

GLOSSARY

acquaintance rape sexual intercourse without consent when the victim knows the aggressor personally; involves the use of force, intimidation, or deception

adolescence the period of physical and psychological development between childhood and maturity

adrenal gland a gland found in both kidneys; divided into two portions: the adrenal cortex, which produces aldosterone, cortisol, and other hormones serving metabolic functions; and the adrenal medulla, which produces adrenaline and noradrenaline, hormones that help the body combat stress

AIDS acquired immune deficiency syndrome; an acquired defect in the immune system caused by a virus (HIV) and spread by blood or sexual contact; leaves people vulnerable to certain, often fatal, infections and cancers

androgen sex hormone, such as testosterone, produced in the testes of the male and in the adrenal glands of both men and women

anorexia nervosa an eating disorder characterized by an obsession with thinness and by loss of appetite; results in extreme weight loss

bulimia an eating disorder characterized by frequent binging and then purging of food

endocrine system the system of glands located throughout the body that produces hormones and secretes them directly into the bloodstream; plays a key role in growth, reproduction, metabolism, and immune system actions

estrogen a hormone produced in the adrenal glands of both sexes, in the ovaries of women, and in the placentas of fetuses; partially responsible for the development of female secondary sex characteristics

gland a bodily structure that secretes a substance, especially one it has extracted from the blood and altered for subsequent secretion

gonads sexual organs; ovaries or testes

growth spurt a period of rapid development that occurs at the onset of puberty; caused primarily by a growth hormone released from the pituitary gland

hormone a product of the endocrine glands that circulates freely throughout the bloodstream, controlling and regulating other glands and organs by chemical stimulation; directly responsible for the physical changes that occur during puberty

hypothalamus the section of the brain that stimulates the adrenal, pituitary, and thyroid glands; regulates survival processes, such as reproduction, nourishment, and self-defense, by initiating the appropriate physical response through nerve impulses and chemical messengers

identity crisis a strong sense of alienation from both self and society; frequently occurs during adolescence in conjunction with the processes of separation from family and establishment of one's own identity

menarche onset of the menstrual period; signals the midpoint of puberty in females

menstruation the cyclic shedding of the uterine lining that occurs in the absence of pregnancy during the reproductive period (puberty through menopause) of the female

Pap smear a gynecological test administered for the detection and diagnosis of various conditions, particularly cervical cancer

pituitary gland the "master gland"; a small gland located in the brain, attached to the hypothalamus, and composed of two sections: the anterior lobe and the posterior lobe; controls the thyroid, adrenal, and sex glands

primary sex characteristics the physical characteristics that differentiate females and males and are directly involved in reproduction; the female's ability to become pregnant and bear children, the male's ability to impregnate a woman

progesterone a hormone released by the adrenal cortex, corpus luteum, and placenta; more abundant in females than in males; stimulates breast development and prepares the uterus to receive a fertilized egg

puberty the period of rapid growth during which secondary sex characteristics develop and the capability of sexual reproduction is attained; its onset, which is stimulated by a sudden increase in the production of sex hormones, generally occurs in females between the ages of 8 and 14 and in males during their early teens

secondary sex characteristics visible physical characteristics that emerge during puberty and are not directly involved in reproduction; include growth of facial and pubic hair and deepening of voice in males, growth of pubic hair and development of breasts in females

semenarche the first ejaculation; signals the midpoint of puberty in males

sexually transmitted disease STD; any of a group of diseases transmitted through anal or vaginal intercourse; includes AIDS, herpes simplex II, gonorrhea, chlamydia, and syphilis

socialization the process of learning how to interact with others in a given environment; the method by which an individual adapts to the needs of society

social literacy the knowledge of acceptable norms of behavior that enable an individual to get along in society; varies from culture to culture

Sturm und Drang "storm and stress"; a German phrase frequently used by psychologists to describe the moodiness that usually accompanies adolescence

testosterone hormone produced in the testes of males and in the adrenal glands of both males and females; responsible for the development of male secondary sex characteristics

thyroid a glandular structure located at the base of the neck; regulates growth and many of the metabolic processes

PICTURE CREDITS

INDEX

Acne, 34
Acquaintance rape, 70–72
Acquired immune deficiency syn-drome (AIDS), 69–70
Adolescence
  alienation, 46
  conflicts, 20, 22, 45–46, 56
  definitions, 22–24
  differences among individuals, 24, 26, 33, 37
  differences between sexes, 26–33. *See also* Gender
  education, 16–17, 69, 79–82
  emotional development, 37, 44–50, 55, 72, 74, 77–78
    coping strategies, 49–50
  emotional turmoil, 18–20, 22, 47–49, 56
  family and, 47–48, 54–59, 71, 74, 77–80, 84
  history of, 15–19, 29
  identity, 42–43, 45–47, 51, 53–60, 67, 71, 75–76
  intellectual development, 37–44, 48, 55, 62, 81–82
  internationally, 82–84
  models for, 53–54, 58
  negative body image, 33–35, 74
  onset, 26, 28–29, 31, 35
  in other cultures, 21–22, 82–84
  physical changes, 22, 25–35, 48, 72
    breast development, 25, 28
    growth, 25–26, 29–33, 35
  poverty, 69, 79–84
  rebellion, 57–58, 67
  roles, 22, 45, 53–54, 74, 79
  self-consciousness, 42–43
  and society, 21, 44–45, 72, 74, 81–82, 84
  socioeconomic factors, 57–58, 77–81
  study of, 19, 21. *See also specific studies*

Adolescence (Hall), 19
Adolescence and Individuality (Gallatin), 47
Adolescence magazine, 34, 56–58
"Adolescent Development and the Onset of Drinking" (Jessor), 66–67
Adolescents Today (Dacey), 34
Adrenal gland, 26
Africa, 82, 84
Ageton, Suzanne S., 70
Alcohol, 66–67, 71–72, 79
Androgens, 31
Anorexia nervosa, 35
Aristotle, 16
Asia, 82–83
Autonomy, 23, 35–36, 45, 55, 58–59, 67, 74, 77–80

Balswick, J. O., 57
Behavioral influences, 54. *See also* Stereotypes
Behavioral Research Institute, 70
Benedict, Ruth, 22
Birth control, 43, 68–69
Blum, Robert, 68
Bulimia, 35
Byron, Lord, 18

Child labor, 16–17
"Chitling test," 82
Chlamydia, 70
Colorado Journal of Educational Research, 41
Coming of Age in Samoa (Mead), 22
Contemporary Issues in Adolescent Development (Conger), 58
Cox, Frank, 66
Creativity, 43, 56, 60
Cultural anthropology, 21–22
Curtis, Russell, 57–58

Rebecca Stefoff is a Philadelphia-based author and editor who has written more than 25 nonfiction books, many of them for young-adult readers. She holds a Ph.D. in English from the University of Pennsylvania, where she taught from 1974 to 1977. She recently completed a two-year term as editor in chief of *TLC*, a health-oriented magazine for hospital inpatients.

Dale C. Garell, M.D., is medical director of California Children Services, Department of Health Services, County of Los Angeles. He is also associate dean for curriculum at the University of Southern California School of Medicine and clinical professor in the Department of Pediatrics & Family Medicine at the University of Southern California School of Medicine. From 1963 to 1974, he was medical director of the Division of Adolescent Medicine at Children's Hospital in Los Angeles. Dr. Garell has served as president of the Society for Adolescent Medicine, chairman of the youth committee of the American Academy of Pediatrics, and as a forum member of the White House Conference on Children (1970) and White House Conference on Youth (1971). He has also been a member of the editorial board of the *American Journal of Diseases of Children*.

C. Everett Koop, M.D., Sc.D., is former Surgeon General, Deputy Assistant Secretary for Health, and Director of the Office of International Health of the U.S. Public Health Service. A pediatric surgeon with an international reputation, he was previously surgeon-in-chief of Children's Hospital of Philadelphia and professor of pediatric surgery and pediatrics at the University of Pennsylvania. Dr. Koop is the author of more than 175 articles and books on the practice of medicine. He has served as surgery editor of the *Journal of Clinical Pediatrics* and editor-in-chief of the *Journal of Pediatric Surgery*, Dr. Koop has received nine honorary degrees and numerous other awards, including the Denis Brown Gold Medal of the British Association of Paediatric Surgeons, the William E. Ladd Gold Medal of the American Academy of Pediatrics, and the Copernicus Medal of the Surgical Society of Poland. He is a Chevalier of the French Legion of Honor and a member of the Royal College of Surgeons, London.